EMOTIONAL INCEST

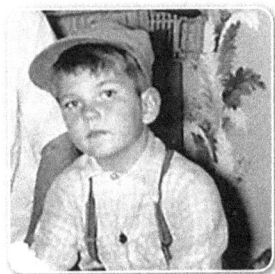

A Childhood Stolen

JIM GORDON PH. D

Paperback: 978-1-965632-29-1
eBook: 978-1-965632-30-7
Library of Congress Control Number: 2024920469

Ordering Information:

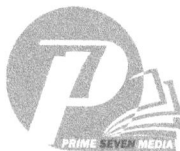

Prime Seven Media
518 Landmann St.
Tomah City, WI 54660

Printed in the United States of America

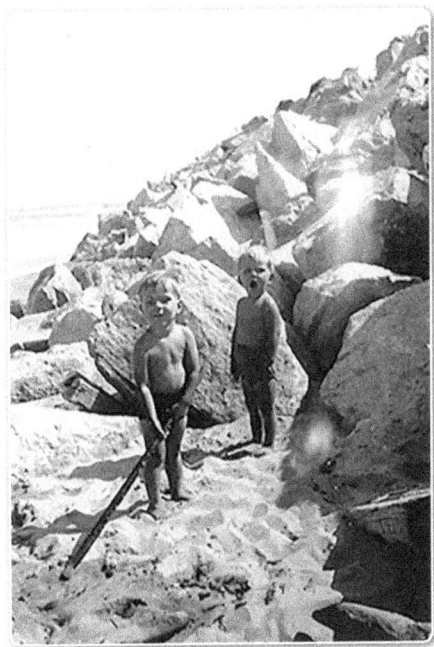

"Shrinks often go into this field
to work out their own problems, then
they get a real job later on"
dr g

dedicated to-
Anne, Matt, Danny,
Carol, Cam, Cate, Christy,
Cody, Ariana, Fred,
God, Kate, Kevin, Sergey,
Aunt Lil, Aunt Helen
and Ross
for listening to
all my 'thoughts' about this issue
for the past umpteen years....
and
the rest of my extended family support group
for hangin' in there,
listening
AND
NOT hangin' me!!!

...

Dear Reader,

Many years ago, when I was on staff in an STD (Sexually Transmitted Disease) Clinic, we would remind folks who came in to test, that when you are sleeping with someone, you are not just sleeping with that person at the moment, but everyone that person had already slept with! They would be carrying whatever viruses and STD's they might have picked up along the way!

Well, guess what? The same is true psychologically and emotionally. When you are dating someone, living with them, marrying them, you are not just dealing with that person but everyone they have dealt with in the past. They will react to you in many ways based on their past experiences and traumas with someone like you who is there for them at the moment.

To better understand the reactions and personalities of folks you deal with, I highly recommend reading about many different types of folks and their issues as it will help in relationships to realize there are many stories in folks, not always excuses for crappy attitude, but certainly often reasons! For instance, on the surface and for folks who meet me, up front they think I'm a mellow person, easy going but... inside I'm a frustrated angst ridden soul.

This book is an in-depth look at one type of harmful experience - Emotional Incest - that shapes the actions and reactions of those who have lived it. When armed with knowledge about this phenomenon, you will be able to more easily recognize the signs in others who have lived it. You will be able to better understand why they behave as they do and the reasons why they relate to you as they do. Understanding builds empathy, which helps us to strengthen – or end – relationships as we care for ourselves and others. Without understanding whats going on, we aren't well-equipped to make such important relationship decisions. I hope to add fodder to your awareness reserve in your head and help you be more fully-equipped! My alternative titles for the book are **"LIFE, LIBERTY and the PURSUIT OF ANGER"** and "Alcoholic Mothers never die, they lie in their Grave waiting for you". You will understand those titles too as you read on.

As you go through this book, use whatever works for you, and try to listen to some of the other stuff too. Glean anything that might help you personally or help you understand others around you, and "bank" the rest for later. You never know what might be useful at another later time in your life. In my case, I may have been denied the chance to "be a little boy", at least at the appropriate chronological time in my life, i.e., when I WAS a little boy, but now as an older guy, I've found that it is truly never toooooo late to have a happy childhood!

As you read my book, I'll explain what EMOTIONAL INCEST is. It is not a well known issue. Then we'll spend time on my own story. Yup, "it's all about me" for those chapters. But not really, my story about shows how life deals us stuff and how we - you and I - can handle it well and efficiently, with grace and class... or not! We can all learn from each other, that's why group process works so well. You'll learn how I handled what life dealt me, from the crazy stuff I experienced, as well as the good stuff, and see how one person (dr. g!) handled some really odd situations. Or parts of my life where I just took a different path than others.

You'll see how those experiences and my reactions to them brought me to the place I am today. They developed my character, parts of which you will like and parts of which I'm sure you'll not like. But no one will say that I don't have character, a personality of my own, or that I'm bland! "Intensely mellow" is how I describe myself – an oxymoron, I know – but befitting as you get to know me.

I'll also share true stories based on my professional life as a psychotherapist in Beverly Hills. They take place every day and night in Beverly Hills and West Hollywood, the cities of celebs with Oscars, losers with broken dreams, the homeless guy "with a script out there," confused lonely millionaires, wanna-be's and hangers-on, has-beens and one-hit-wonders, mansions, limos, drugs, silicon, vaping, narcissism and.... dysfunction and depression!!! You'll see a story or two about the folks from the desert where I was on staff at a stroke rehab unit for years, as well as my experiences teaching at an all-female Catholic University in Brentwood/Los Angeles.

Along the way, you'll get to know some of the folks who work in my office as therapists, counselors, interns, colleagues and who are "here to help you solve your problems, guide you through your life, find your true self". We'll tackle tough questions such as, "Can we really do that?" and "Are we more messed up than our patients?" You'll hear about my cop friends, entertainment buddies, colorful clients and characters who are either patients or acquaintances or just folks I've met on the street, but have interesting stories. And you'll hear about those I call the "pre-dead," mere place holders in life who are breathing yes, existing yes, but just barely.

It's quite entertaining – if sad – because, as you might imagine, many folks in LA are ideal "poster children" for the Diagnostic Manual of Psychological Disorders. I'll share some of their lives, both the bright and the dark sides. Under the makeup, behind the key-guarded driveway gates, underneath their degrees and titles, behind the badge, they have the same issues as Mr. and Mrs. Average American. Hear what they feel, what they think, how they live. Most importantly, you'll learn how they destroy themselves and make attempts to recover and rebuild.

I'm real. The others - the people on both sides of the couch and the law – that I present are composites due to confidentiality issues - but every story is very real! So sit back, get comfortable, read on and listen to learn. Remember, your life is a precious gift. Don't waste it. It's the only one you'll get.

And like our lives, this book is a "work in progress" with more things to come and updates to add in the future. Please feel free to email me at my office, bhcounseling@gmail.com to chat if you have some thoughts from your adventure or questions. I also have a YouTube channel where you can hop on and ask or SHARE YOUR STORY... my tube site is: **@DrG90212** You can also add to my Emotional-incest.com website if you want to add your story.

Thanks for reading, and I hope I can help make your journey a little better

dr g
b.hills, ca 2024

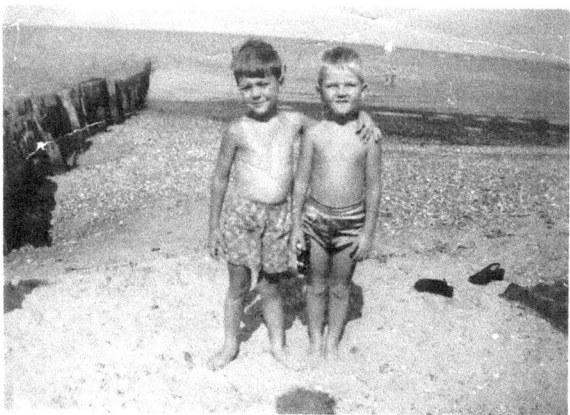

Table of Contents

  b. Ross, my first 'healthy parent'

  c. My Legacy- MSMU, groups, books, chats

 3. Offices, jobs - decision points

  a. Reminder of why Shrinks "Shrink"

  b. Sorting things out

  c. My Counselors and Staff

 A. Reflections on Life, Death, 'the Journey'

  1. It's never too late for a happy childhood

 B. Reparenting/Surrogate Parents

 C. Healing Resources

Alternate title: "Life, Liberty and the Pursuit of Anger" defined: **Liberty**, is the freeing of one's self from the bondage to that parent, and then dealing with your **Anger**, repressed and overt, that Emotional Incest has caused but now having a healthier **LIFE**.

PART ONE

What is Emotional Incest?

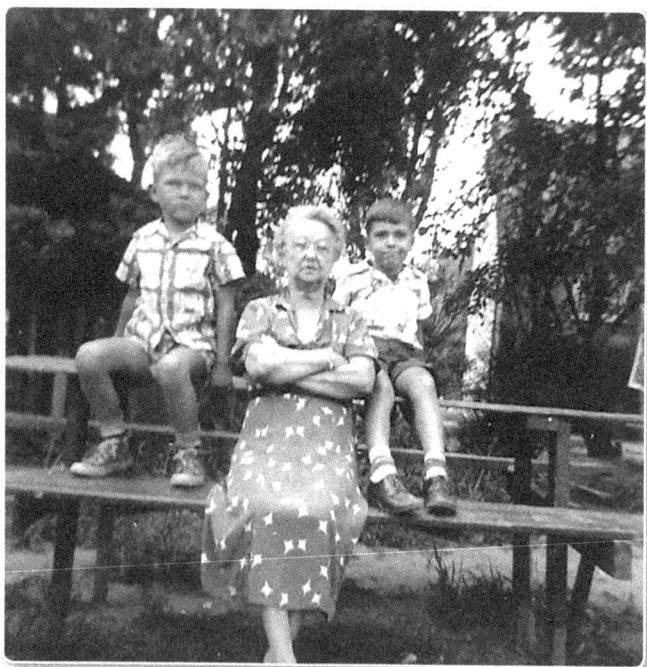

I. What is Emotional Incest?

A. Defining and Identifying Emotional Incest

The term Emotional Incest (also known as: covert incest; psychic incest; covert relationships) describes a relationship that exists between a parent and a child that is sexualized without actual physical incest/sexual contact. The relationships are harmful and one-sided, and similar to a relationship between adult sexual partners but without the type of physical contact that would qualify it as child sexual abuse. The long term effects are similar to, though less severe, than that of sexual incest.

The definition of Emotional Incest has a broad set of criteria. Basically, Emotional Incest is a covert incest. It is a form of emotional abuse in which the relationship between a parent and a child is inappropriately sexualized without actual sexual contact. Often substance abuse is associated with covert incest, as seen via the alcoholic dependent needy dysfunctional parent for instance. The effects of covert incest somewhat mimic sexual incest but to a lesser degree. The victims have been described as having anger or guilt towards parents and have issues with self-esteem, addiction as well as sexual and emotional intimacy and thus evolved this book.

B. Why it matters and why I write about it

Emotional Incest started to be recognized and acknowledged about 25 to 30 years ago. It has primarily been defined by the few researchers and therapists who acknowledge it and work with it, as an emotionally abusive relationship between a parent (or step-parent) and child that does not involve incest or sexual intercourse. It involves similar interpersonal dynamics that are much like the relationship between married or unmarried sexual partners. The dynamics of the relationship is particularly similar to 'old time' seasoned partners who have gotten comfortable with each other over the years - marriages where sex is no longer the prime purpose in their lives, but the emotional support and bond is strong between the members of the relationship.

Think of the couple that has been married for many years, sex has waned, or is non-existent, but they still rely on each other, and at times need each other, for support in their daily lives. An example, is that alcoholic mom who struggles with daily life and functioning, who is often put down by her spouse for being a drunk, but she pulls aside 'Jr', who has just celebrated his 8th birthday, and talks to him, reminding him what a bastard his dad is, but that only he (Jr) really understands her, and she can only go on living thanks to Jr. and thanks to Jr. being there for her! Jr. is reminded "don't you ever treat your wife the way your dad treats me, Jr. I love you and you are my life". Now 'Jr' is hooked, seduced emotionally yet has found himself into a position of power without realizing it which I'll explain later. In a sense Jr. now has a case load! And often for the rest of his life, having to take care of mom's emotional needs.

Emotional Incest is a parent responding to a child's love with adult sexuality and energy but without physical sexual activity. Relationship problems between parents often facilitate emotional incest; as the parents distance themselves from each other both physically, sexually, and emotionally, one parent then begins focusing more and more on his or her child. The child becomes the surrogate partner and source of emotional support for the parent. The abusing parent may also be afraid or unable to meet their needs through a relationship with another adult. Alcohol and other substance addictions are often present in emotional incest situations.

Emotional Incest rears up when a parent is unable or unwilling to maintain a relationship, healthy or otherwise, with another adult and forces that emotional role of a spouse onto their child instead. The child's needs are ignored and instead the relationship exists and focuses primarily to meet the needs of the parent.

The adult usually is not aware of the issues created by their actions, and justifies the relationship in a variety of ways. Emotional incest happens when parents fill their own inner emptiness by overly connecting with their child, bonding as equals and "buddies". A red flag is the mom who tells her daughter that they are like 'sisters' not like parent and child, they both tend to see this as a wonderful healthy thing. However, parents need to learn how to take responsibility for their own feelings so that their children do not feel and experience this surreptitious maneuver. I often use the words premeditated and non-premeditated in dealing with cases where it needs to be decided if someone is purposely out to hurt or injure someone, of it is happens in the midst of other issues.

In Emotional Incest, seldom has the parent intentionally said to themselves, "I'm gonna screw up my kid's life, because I am angry and want to hurt them." That would be premeditated, with the goal to hurt, get back at, or damage someone on purpose. No, Emotional Incest, is normally non- premeditated and is purviewed to be doing each other good, doing a favor for each other in a helping way. Friends will often say how lucky you are to have your kid be so close to you, so supportive. The kid will hear from folks how great it is that they are so "there for mom" or dad... They will all feel good.

Mom's hugs and but lots of attention to Jr. can become weird after time. All young boys reach a point where mom's hug is 'gross' BUT that is normal child development. It's when mom continues to hug and hug... and yup, hug some more with an odd energy that is felt by the kid, that starts to feel odd, but he can't express what is wrong with it. And the child has to be in an adult role and miss out their childhood often. Later on I refer to "I was Never a Little Boy". I was an Adult at 6. So today, I often remind folks that it is NEVER TO LATE for a happy childhood. But we'll get back to that later...

Early on, the affected young person can experience distress in their own personal friendships and relationships and later on, in their sexual relationships. Mom's often become jealous of the child's friends, and makes the child feel guilty when he or she does not spend time with mom but goes off with kid friends. Often, mom's will have some very disparaging comments about the child's friends, or make some comments after the kid's friends are over to the house that makes it clear mom does not want the kids around. Then the choice is, "do I hang with my friends, or do I hurt my mom?" Tough call for many kids who are torn between 'loving mom who needs me' and having fun with my friends. Difficult decision at times.

And this is one of those times when being mom's best friend can become a perk. The perks of staying with the parent, gives the kid special privileges and rank in the family. And if there are other kids, the chosen one will have earned that rank over his or her siblings by being loyal to mom. As my friend Valentin stated once, "support becomes a product", i.e., "if you give me support, you will earn a tangible reward" which with Emotional Incest kids can range from earning the use of the family car when older, to loans and to outright dollar gifts. It is a form of covert power and control. The child ends up with some unwanted power over the other siblings, or over the spouse of the seductive parent. For instance, dad might come home and say to Mom and 'her kid', "Do whatever you want, whatever I want doesn't matter here anymore, you two seem to make all the decisions around here anyway." Something my father used often!

Moms mess up when out of the clear blue, they sit you down on the couch, grab your arms, look intently into your eyes, and tell you how much they love you, and how important you are to her. It's a creepy feeling, but the beginning of the destruction. Kids don't know exactly how to describe what is felt.

Dads can do the same, more so with daughters than their sons, though, alcoholic dads seem very prone to latch on to a son, reminding them they want the kid to be everything the drunk dad isn't. When dad's had a drink or twenty, that bond usually goes like this, "'son, your dad's a drunk, I'm so sorry, but you are smart, you can make it, you are the most important person in my world, I want to see you succeed, to have everything I didn't. You give me reason to live, and keep living." Now, Jr. has a case load and 24/7 job with Dad. Dad may be successful at business, or even socially, but Jr. is privy to dads inner pain and has to make dad happy and becomes responsible for that happiness.

Emotional Incest occurs when a parent sucks dry a child to fill their own inner emptiness that is really the parent's responsibility to fill, not the kids. Kids are not born to be, nor did they sign on at birth, as cruise director and therapist for mom or dad! Dad and Mom are supposed to give the kid energy, not suck them dry. When a parent abandons himself or herself emotionally and gives up on their future, that parent then latches on to the kid to fill the chasm that occurs from self-abandonment. While it might not be as traumatic as sexual incest, it occurs for the same reasons - a wounded parent using a child addictively to get love and avoid their own emptiness and pain. Robbing the kid of their childhood.

Emotional incest parents often feel they are being good dads and moms, or will even often call themselves 'super parents' when they spend lots of time talking with their kids. They might follow them into their rooms at night and visit, go for many ride in the car to 'talk', dine out lots with the child. YES, some of that is fine, but with emotional incest parents, the talk becomes focused on the parent venting about their issues and the kid is getting nothing but tired! And drained. The parent child role gets reversed with the kid becoming the parent, listening to their child (mom or dad) sort things out. Again, occasionally that is fine and growth for both, but not if it is taking the place of adult interaction.

A parent with a gaping inner hole that comes from inner abandonment cannot just stop the emotional incest without recognizing what is going on, they don't feel it, or see it as hard on the kid. They need help in finding healthy sources or resources to nurture themselves and not put the weight of THEIR world onto the child's little shoulders. Ironically, one of the perks for the kid, is that weight does bring a shift in power, the kid starts feeling that they are strong, that they are powerful, that they are good kids because they can and do handle the problems of mom or dad.

And dang, guess what? Many of them become ... therapists, or social workers, without realizing part of that choice is to sort themselves out. They become Adult Children, and are the ones in the psych class who say they chose to become therapists and social workers, because they are good listeners and have been told how helpful they are by others. Certainly a parent can stop the overt actions, but to stop the energetic pull, they need to be doing their own inner work so they can learn to fill their own inner emptiness and not rely on their kids.

I mention the term Adult Children. In the world of alcoholism, the Adult Child of Alcoholics is a well known situation. Where the child has to handle issues around home, because mom or dad are often too drunk to deal with the issues. I also suggest that alcoholic parents can play a role in the emotional incest. And for just those reasons, the kid becomes responsible for their younger siblings, or dealing with relatives, or even running some small businesses if the parent is not capable due to alcohol or substance abuse. The kid might be the one who has to call dad's work and explain 'dad was bitten by a spider and won't be at work today' when of course, dad is just drunk or hung over. But the kid again has to be thrust into the adult world and deal with things mom or dad should be handling.

Years ago, one of my clients had to deal with his dad having a drinking problem, and dad also would often hook up with ladies from the bar. He would call his son, Jon, and tell him he was gonna be late, and "you know son, what that means, so take care of it." Meaning, that Jon was now responsible at 14 to find a good excuse for mom to understand why dad was not home, and to be ready to keep mom happy in dad's absence - take her to dinner or movie to keep her mind off dad's absence, and often, then to be nursemaid to dad when he did come home wasted at 3 am and needed help sobering up.

The term Adult Child is a good one for both situations, the child of an alcoholic and the child in the emotional incest world. Both have to be the 'adult' in their situation, and as shown, many emotional incest situations are based around alcohol issues (or other substance issues) of the parent.

You might be asking, "If this book is about Emotional Incest, why did you originally consider the title 'Life, Liberty, and the Pursuit of Anger'?" Here's the why - We are 'given' a life at birth. We are given opportunities to grow and liberate ourselves and become the best person we can be. Normally we are given a parent or two who are supposed to be our tour-guide to Life. Who is supposed to be there for us. To do their best to help us get to a healthy adulthood.

Sometimes that gets screwed up. And some of these survivors deal with the detours in life better than others. Some just blame everyone else and get mad at the world. To understand better the world of Emotional Incest Survivors, we will talk about actual lives, from my own experience of 'Never having been a little boy', always the adult from 6 years old on to the stories I talk about and share, who will never grow up without some boundaries and awareness. In the next section of my book, I'll talk about how you can free yourself, liberate what's inside of you to make you the best person you can be, and free yourself from the anger and frustration that is often not recognized in emotional incest kids, but for now just listen to the comments I make and suggestions as I SURVIVE, and get re-born not in a Christian Religion style but in actual day to day life. Others see it, and feel it, but the kids themselves often don't. After all, they think that the lives they are/were living is the norm in the first place. And then there were some perks and freedoms afforded them due to the closeness with their parent. Plus, they have been told how special and wonderful they are by one of the adults in their lives, so how could they not believe they are happy and things are wonderful?

But, there is underlying anger, in ways unknown to the child as the child is enjoying staying home from school a lot with mom, having a few drinks with dad even though they are just a teen, getting privileges other kids aren't getting. It sees so perfect at the time. However, inside the kid, they sorta realize over time that they were 'used and abused' rather than just nurtured. Angry sometimes as the other parent or relatives for not jumping in and protecting their childhood time.

Anger is something we all have, it is a normal emotion but don't want to acknowledge it, or be labeled as and Angry person.

◻ ◻ ◻ ◻

Why do we get to these situations? What brings us to dysfunction? Or psych issues that manifest and grow? How about the kids who have been physically, sexually, incestuously abused vs those with Emotional Incest? And, is it possible that everybody really is screwed emotionally up anyway? Are these issues really our parents fault? Or are they society's fault? Maybe the school system's is the failure? Can we blame the church? Who do we blame? Must we blame? Do we need to have a scapegoat?

Or do we ask questions, look inside, so we can get a handle on life and on what makes us all tick? In this book, we'll look at some of this. Lots of times we are just looking for that excuse, or any excuse to blame others for everything. Turning ourselves into "Victims of Life" so we don't have to be responsible.

I have a T-shirt that says, "to Err is human, to be able to blame it on someone else shows good Management Potential". I also remind folks that often there are reasons for doing things, for feeling certain ways or taking certain actions, but these are not excuses. For instance, in Los Angeles, being late for something due to traffic is not usually a good excuse because we all know about LA traffic and its unpredictability! So too bad if it's the reason you were late, you know the traffic issue so you should allow for it. So much for the excuse part.

I apologize for some of the rambling dialogue in the book, but my reason is that there have been very few books written about this issue, and that it has been a hidden issue, so I shall use that as my "excuse" for tossing in things here and there vs a totally organized predictably written book! Excuses, excuses, excuses... Hell, I'm still working out my issues as I write this and think.

BTW, here's a perfect time to throw this point out to you - in my domestic violence program I'm always reminding people there are reasons versus excuses and that they are not always the same thing. Years ago Oprah Winfrey had a mom on her TV show who had been stuck sitting in a court case hearing and listen as a man talked about sexually abusing her son who was 11 years old. The man described the pleasure he had as well as the pleasure the child seemed to be having as he was engaging in sex with the boy as a defense for what he did. The mother was very enraged, and the next day came to court with a gun, shot and killed the perpetrator as he was pleading his case in the courthouse. Her actions initiated of course, much of our nowadays having to be screened for weapons when we go to courts and other situations. However, as Oprah pointed out, did the mom have a good reason for wanting to kill this guy? Certainly. But it didn't give her a legal 'excuse' to go ahead and kill him. Unfortunately the mom had to pay the penalty for murdering him.

When we're driving in traffic if somebody is being a jerk in the front of us in traffic, we have a reason to be angry with that person for messing things up in traffic, slowing us down, but it's not really an excuse to go ahead, grab the Glock 9 you have on your dashboard and shoot and kill them! **REASONS, are not always EXCUSES!!**

I am not trying to excuse the behavior of folks who are emotional incest survivors, but just trying to enlighten the world to an issue, another dirty little secret that gets swept under the rug most of the time. For many of the clients I talk to who have these Emotional Incest issues, they thought they were the only one experiencing what was happening. They had heard that parents are never wrong from their churches, cultures and from the parents themselves.

They often felt isolated, and remember, many parents in these cases don't want the kids to have friends since the parent wants the full attention.

We can't go back and assuage everyone who has struggled with this issue or similar ones. But we can probe and think and sort things out together. Hopefully by the last page of the book, we will both know more about the issue of emotional incest, about ourselves, and about others and have a better handle on Life itself. And help folks become aware of these situations and maybe change how they deal with their kids before they totally damage them.

As a therapist I had one of those experiences I mention to my students who are going into the therapy field, that as you hear a patient/client tell you about their life drama you often either get uncomfortable, or ironically relieved as you hear a story they are telling that parallels YOUR life. My friend Aaron had that happen as he was listening to the play TOMMY, and when they get to the part where we hear that Tommy had been 'fiddled and fiddled' by his uncle (as in sexually abused), Aaron totally connected to it emotionally and realized what he had hidden for years. And my therapy intern Aimee who I mention elsewhere in the book, was working with a 12 year old girl when the girl described being sexually manipulated by her grandfather. Aimee listened and listened to the story, then stepped out of the session saying to the girl that she needed to use the restroom. Instead, she came to my office in tears, as she described how she now realized her father had done exactly the same acts with her. Aimee broke down and cried to me, and said I now realize WHY I have been so hiding from things all my life, why I avoided talking about things and now realize why I want to help others to get through what I had avoided.

The part of the original book title, ... "and Pursuit of Anger" is based on my life hearing and realizing at an older age, in my 40's, that I had been Emotionally Abused as I listened to a patient of mine, Josiah. As mentioned later in this tome (book about heavy subjects!), my mother had been abandoned by her father at birth. She imagined her father to be everything he wasn't as she grew up, she was sure that he loved her, missed her, cared about her every day. It was back in the early 1900's, so her communication tools were sending him handwritten letters, hand written pictures for holidays, etc. He was paying alimony from the time she was born. She dreamed of the day she would meet him face to face and hug and hold him and tell him how much she loved him. She 'knew' he missed her. When she was about 18 she got a relative to drive her from home in New Jersey to California to see her 'loving father' where he moved shortly after she was born. She knocked on his door in Long Beach, California and said to the man who opened the door, "I'm Marian, your daughter, I love you and came to see you." His response, "Get away, you are DEAD in my mind, I have supported your mother with alimony, go away or I will call the police". NOT THE RESPONSE my mother had wanted nor dreamed of for her first 18 years of life. Devastated that day, it changed her Life!

She never owned it, but she now needed to get married to a man who she could 'get back at' like her father, and then have a child (me) who could be the one person she could love and who would love her forever. And EVER! Yes, she married a man about 15 years older than she was, she was 26, he was 41. She was perky, a dancer, sexy looking and fun. He was a mentally gifted, serious, book nerd type. Handsome and striking but due to his own issues, very serious about everything. Seldom laughed, had a reasons to be mad at the world which he acted on forever. He used to pound on the kitchen counter when drinking his coffee and complain about politics, the world, and all, every morning as he would get ready for work, or even just for life that day. She did NOT realize that she did this, it was not pre-meditated but just 'happened' and led to more issues for her, for my father and for me.

SO, Josiah was my patient, remember I had not really wanted to be a psychotherapist, but got 'stuck' in this career due to life shifts when Life gives you a detour for many different reasons. I'm sitting there listening to Josiah in his 30's ramble on about his mother and father - yeah, normal psychotherapy session talks about 'my mother said this...' and 'my father just drank and avoided us...' AND wham it hit me.

Josiah's mother manipulated his life so that he was STUCK with her! And couldn't leave. She did some horrible stuff that he wasn't angry about, just saying she was sick. But as his therapist listening to the things, I was angry. Later realizing some of the same things had happened in my world, my life. Damn.

So why it matters and why I treat it & write about it, let's talk... why care about or be interested in Emotional Incest stuff when there are kids out there who have other heavy problems like autism, deafness or cancer?

I may look like a little boy in the picture on the cover, but I was already an old man inside. One author wrote an article some time ago, titled 'why man invented god'. The premise was that we need to have answers. When things don't go the way we might like we want answers, reasons, to make things right with our minds. For instance, when a sweet young kid gets hit by a car and dies at age 10, we need to have an answer in some form or another to the tragedy. Logic at that time fails us, and to write it off using the adage, that in everything there is a lesson, still leaves the kid dead, parents grieving and lots of unanswered questions. BUT, then we turn to 'god' for the answer, because "God, he or she, must have had a reason to do this, and to take this kid 'to heaven' at such a young age." Some would say, that kid must have been very special that god wanted him or her so early. Or that somewhere there is a meaning for this, and that god knows why even though we don't. God makes no mistakes, we've been told and indoctrinated to believe that. So, now that we have turned over the irrational death to god, we can rest, and sleep and eventually be at peace. For many of us, no we would not just accept it, but...

Well, back to the little kid on the cover, yeah me, I don't understand yet, 60 years later why I was given this 'gift' of being an 'adult child of alcoholics'. Was it a gift? Was it just a liability, or was it a joke by god! For many of us, our childhood has been stealthily stolen. Later in our lives, we start to think about what we missed, and why, and then mourn the childhood from which we were deprived. Some of my patients who are the most angry or depressed in adulthood are finding that it had its roots in their never having been a kid, in having had to be an adult during their childhood years. Or never treated appropriately as a kid. Sometimes major depression sets in, often feeling defeated forever. Sad time.

In losing our 'kidhood' to emotional incest, we end up switching roles with mom, dad or both. And later when you realize this, can you bring yourself to divorce your mom and/or Dad without guilt? Can you stay away from them knowing the damage that was done, but not feel that you have to be there because as you have been told many times, "you have to love her because she is your mom"! Or "he is your dad. You owe it to him."

There is an old adage, "sticks and stones will break my bones, but names will never hurt me." Boy is that one ever wrong. Thanks to those 'words', therapists have careers!! And bars and breweries have good businesses. Yup, broken bones can be healed, set and repaired in the emergency room, but 'words' can and will eat at you forever!... and ever... and...ever! Oh yeah, and FOREVER!

To understand this issue, Emotional Incest, I'm inviting you to share in my journey... My journey to SELF, and I will share some things from the other folks I've worked with who have this issue. I'll whine about, what I've experienced up to now, what I've learned and where I'm hoping to head. What I will hope is that I've left for the world is my legacy so far, and what I'd like to add to that legacy before I expire. I feel we all need to leave a legacy, not just offering our daily presence on this earth in day to day humdrum which happens just by our mere existence, or as some do, having their legacy be a building named after them, or those whose legacy is that they own lots of expensive toys?

Rather, I feel a major part of a good healthy legacy is living life gracefully, managing life with dignity and class while leaving behind some new awareness of things that will help those growing up today. Helping folks find ways of dealing with the speed bumps in the Journey of Life, by humbly leaving a legacy that has impacted some folks for them to have a better life thanks to my time on this earth.

❑ ❑ ❑ ❑

When I started working on the book and looked into things, EMOTIONAL INCEST was not an acknowledged issue or even defined. To this day, it is not a DSM 5 item (the DIAGNOSTIC and STATISTICAL MANUAL of MENTAL DISORDERS used by Psychiatrists and Psychologists for diagnosis).

If you GOOGLE it you will find comments and resources that did not exist 20 years ago. One site suggests that Emotional Incest is when a parent or primary caregiver treats a child like a romantic partner. The parent relies on the child to get their own emotional needs met that would normally be fulfilled by an adult partner.

They remind us that the relationship is not physically or sexually intimate in nature, but it is still inappropriate and unfair to the child. The kid is placed into an adultlike emotional role with that parent and they become the main emotional support for that person.

Parents often get into topics that a child should not be hearing from mom or dad. These conversations can put a kid in a very uncomfortable position.

There are numerous sites now, one even has a chart of the symptoms of Emotional Incest, and another has a test you can do to see if it is your problem!

PART TWO

Here is My Story - Emotional Incest in Real Life

"Alcoholic Mothers Never Die,
They Just Lie in their Graves
waiting for you..."
dr. g

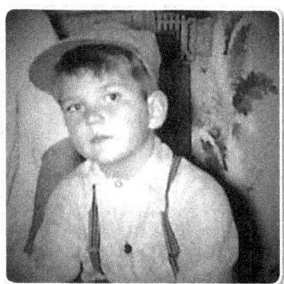

II. Emotional Incest in Real Life

My Story - How I Got here

Setting the stage, let's start talking about the adult me (chronologically at least) in my role of Psychotherapist and Educator and we'll work back through the scenes back to the not so innocent Little Jimmy in the pictures.

Remember, in many ways I was living a lie as you will see in the section after this called "Why Shrinks often Shrink" while I had to find my inner child and let it grow a bit to make me a healthier adult. The lie that I was telling myself was that I was there to HELP others only, but was actually finding my 'SELF', while helping others as I listened to their stories and helped them sort out their drama. I did find myself little by little. The reality of course, is that I did help many sort their lives out too while I was going on my journey. Ironically the word 'lie' I mentioned above plays a bit role in my story too as you will see later in the book, where my mother spread salacious lies to control my life, my growth and my future which also took me 30 years to figure out and deal with by 'divorcing her'.

Some of you may know about Adult Children of Alcoholics. ACOA is discussed from time to time in the book but by the time I was 10 years old, I was in charge of the family, in charge of finding the money to pay the bills, lying to my drunk mother's and dad's bosses about why they didn't make it to work, and to my teachers about why I couldn't be in school or one very creepy sick where I explained to Mr. Ryder, my Sociology teacher, just before lunch time, that "No, my mother wasn't drunk when she came to pick me up, she just forgot to wear a clothes under her raincoat that day!"

And at 11 years of age, I was looking for my mother's hidden booze bottles and prescription drugs. She used something called Miltown in those days - Meprobamate that was approved for use in generalized anxiety disorders in the United States in 1955, classified as a Schedule IV controlled substance because of its potential for abuse and dependency and seldom used today. She had access from using MANY! different pharmacies and doctors in different towns around the Jersey Shore area. I was also busy tracking down my father at the bars on holidays so he could come home, and we could "have the family together" - yeah sure, while I'd be verbally abused by my father for tracking him down and emotionally seduced by my mother, being "her little man" since dad was mostly out of the scene and she didn't know what she'd do without ME...

As I'm prone to do, here is a short aside from the drill of finding dad who usually was at the Matawan Tavern or Log Cabin B&G. The comment in the last

paragraph about tracking my father in bars takes me
back to a Christmas Eve when I was about 6. As usual
my father had worked all day and did not come directly
home. By phoning aroud, my mother found him at
the infamous Matawan Tavern, which on my travels
back East, I discovered only in the last few years was
torn down. Mother, who was quite attractive, called
her friend who was a Sargent in the local police
department in Laurence Harbor where we lived on
the Raritan Bay. Sarge picked her up with little Jimmy
in tow, and we drove to the Tavern to find father. It was
my first ride in a police car, I remember it to this day,
it was a 1950 two door Chevy. We found my father at
the Tavern, his FAV. He was rather drunk, so shouldn't
be driving, so the cop friend drove my fathers van, in
those days they were panel trucks, back to our house
and then my mother drove the cop car with me in the
front seat... Very cool for a little kid. No, I don't think
I got to use the lights and siren or anything, but it was
fun. And the beginning of a life long avocation that
I fulfilled later as a Volunteer with the LA Sheriff's
Depart for 30+ years.

———————>≈<———————

My mother had many reasons for being the way
she was and for needing to have me as her "little man".
I understand them now, and as I was growing up, my
relationship with her seemed 'normal' to me. Now I
realize she had major issues and reason for them.

It was unfortunate that she had had such a weird childhood herself, but in a way, if she hadn't I wouldn't be writing this today! And because of her struggles, her actions while raising me, what I learned and went through... from my cluelessness, which later turned into insight, and an attempt at integration of the education and learning process, because of this "living-in-it education", I can help others and be a good shrink because I've been there! And I don't mean there as in Hackensack, NJ but THERE as in living through emotional crap. Experience beats all the 'book l'arnin' with a big stick. The education from books puts it in perspective and gives you information for your head, the experience of living it though is the real learning and makes it part of you and gets it to your heart and gut.

So, back to my mother's issues, yes over time I found out my mother had been abused emotionally as a kid. I feel sorry for her. Her mother, my grandmother Helen, was one of four girls born to a priest. Father John Parscouta was a Byzantine Catholic priest from Austria. In Europe, the priests could wed back then so they could increase the number of Catholics in the area much like the Mormons have done by allowing a man to have more than one wife so here were more kids ... and Mormons! So he did and made good on that option by marrying Irenka from Russia and having 4 kids, all girls. He, his wife, and 4 little girls headed to America in 1901 to raise their kids. They lived on the East Coast, mostly working with poorer parishes in New Jersey, Pennsylvania and Connecticut. Father

John showed his Austrian roots in his looks and stature, he was often said to look like Pope John 23rd, plus he was an early ecumenical visionary for the church just as Pope John was. Something the church was truly in need of, but not quite ready for in Father John's era. He was outgoing, friendly, well liked. But open to the new world and its ideas.

Because of his marriage and daughters, he got some hard assignments in parishes. But, it was always a kick for him to arrive in a primarily Austrian/Hungarian speaking working class parish, and introduce his wife and daughters. In the United States, the Byzantine priests did not marry, so this did cause a stir. In research, I have found he was ordained in the United States by a Roman Catholic Bishop as was the practice in those days since Byzantine's were limited in this country. So he often help out at Roman Catholic Parishes too, another eye opener and ahead of his time. I have an old picture of him dressed in his vestments (clergy garb) astride a horse in 1920 ready to ride from one parish in Kingston, PA to another for Sunday services.

His wife Irenka was beautiful, so their girls were all very attractive. So attractive that three of them ended up in show business. All were on stage as dancers and known as the "Park Sisters" working with the infamous Ziegfield Follies. Their last name was Parscouta, and in those day everyone made their names simpler and 'more American'. They took the name Parscouta and made it Parks as their last name. My Great Aunt

Blanco, who was the next to the oldest, even had her own starring show, where she was a principal(lead) in a summer show on the roof of the Winter Garden Theater on Broadway. The other two were "just part of their shows". Father John would proudly attend shows with his collar turned around, then confuse and startle folks as he introduced his daughters and brought his collar back around denoting his being clergy after the show!

Those Great-Aunts, Marian, Eve, and Blanco, remained on the stage for only a short run, less than 5 years. Blanco told me she had a motto when dating and doing 'the BROADWAY THING', "Don't give me minks, diamonds and flashy cars, give me stocks, bonds, and negotiables". So, she retired from the biz by age 26, even though she was the most successful in her run. She never had to work again, and died at 87! More about her later.

Great-Aunt Marian also retired young from Broadway and married for a short time to a Cadillac Dealer... But, what a surprise, she had a thing for ... priests. Father issues??? And I mean Father in multiple modes. She had a long term, about 60 years... relationship with a priest! "Same time, next year Marion?" Great-Aunt Marian's lifetime boyfriend Father Arthur was a young fledgling priest in her own dad's parish in Pennsylvania. When he met Marian she was just a teenager. They bonded, and remained in love for 60 years. When she died at 76, I went to the retirement home where she spent her last years to pack her things and clear out her stuff. It was in Corpus Christi, Texas... she was the most religious of the daughter, thus living in Corpus Christi (Body of Christ) was a must for her and she loved to point out the meaning of the city name. While there, I was intrigued as a number of the old folks came up to me and expressed their condolences at her passing. They would tell me that though she was basically a recluse, spending very little time with the neighbors in the building, she must have been a wonderful saintly woman since, the now Monsignor Arthur had come all the way from the East Coast to do the burial service, and being such a good friend, he even paid for her funeral! They were so impressed that this man, who had been a young priest in her life, had kept in touch for so many years... little did they know that for those 60 years, every summer for a few weeks, it was more than just 'keeping in touch'...! I was discreet for once, and did not elucidate the actual details of the relationship!! May they both rest in peace now.

Great-Aunt Eve, the third of the dancing Park Sisters didn't fare so well. Her catholic guilt got to her. Success as a dancer and the seductiveness that went with being a female star/performer was too foreign to her religious beliefs, she felt she was a heathen in God's eyes for her lifestyle, so she slashed her beautiful wrists at 24. Short life, short story.

———— ※ ————

Great-Aunt Blanche (Blanco) however, led quite a life. She was the most successful on stage of the three sisters and stayed part of the Zeigfield Follies for a number of years. As mentioned above, she was a principal in that show on the roof of the Winter Garden Theater. Remember in those days, there was no air conditioning inside, so in the summer they had special late night shows on the roof. She did great, stayed on Broadway for a while.

If you ever watch old movies where the stars would take their dogs into the restaurants and seat them at their tables, in true glorious decadent style, while the servers were fawning over the celeb and her pup, then you saw Blanco's lifestyle. I've seen picture's of Blanco and her Airedale named Buster at one of the finer New York theater area restaurants, Sardi's back in the 1920's. Buster liked steak! And he got it. Yup, seated at the table eating with a well coiffed server, with the classic white towel over one arm, serving them. She hooked up with some big folks and had special stature on Broadway in her day.

Now thanks to the internet, I have done some research into the shows, and found a number of PLAYBILLS of her shows. In some where she was the "principal" of a show, it is very interesting to find names such as 'William C. Fields and William Rogers" as 'part of cast' in her show. YES, well before they became entities on their own, and much beloved by the public.

As I mentioned earlier, Blanco slept around but didn't just do the mink and diamond routine most did.

She did collect well in her ventures, and set herself up financially for life. She retired in her late 20's from show biz and didn't really working again or have to.

She was married for a short time to a Cadillac dealer in the 20's, and enjoyed her cars and golf. She eventually became a ranked golf amateur and went on tour. She fell in love with a ranked tennis player who she planned on marrying. They were quite the couple on the circuit - both cute, young and photogenic. But, one day she went to his place and the police were there. He had gotten busted for being in bed with a minor... A male! So much for that storybook romance.

After his getting busted she stayed away from relationships for a bit, but eventually she hooked up with a married guy who owned a chain of fine jewelry stores on the east coast. He had the bux, she had the body, he had a wife and kids. She also had a few bux of her own saved up from the show days, and lived well in Pelham Manor near New York City. In the fall, Wally (the married guy) would go to Florida with his family. He had a yacht, so he and the family would sail to Florida. He would then send the boat back to pick up Blanco and bring her down for the winter. He put Blanco up in a house in Coral Gables - black maid, new car each year, and an expense account provided of course. My mother got to ride with her aunt Blanco on the boat a number of times, and enjoy the luxury. After 20+ years of this, Blanco got a phone call one day in the mid 50's, "Hi Blanco, my name is Hillary... you and I haven't met, but I know you well. I am Wally's wife.

I want to let you know that Wally died in July. Things will be different this winter in Florida for you. I also want to thank you for providing whatever it was that was missing in our marriage, that you seemed to have provided that kept Wally and I together so we could raise our kids and have a good life. The deed to the house you use in Florida is on the dining table when you get there, the house is yours. There is a new car in the garage, for the last time. I don't want to meet you... ever. Have a good life. Bye."

Later Blanco moved to Hollywood where she connected with old show biz people. She lived in the infamous Garden Court Apartments on Hollywood Boulevard. In its last years, it was sort of a precursor to a motion picture retirement home by housing lots of old, older, and really damn old entertainment people. Perky Blanco even connected there with another guy who did her well, a silent screen giant movie maker, married of course, who found Blanco, who was about 20 years younger than he was at the time. They hit it off. They had fun - wined and dined til he expired. Fun times for both. She did well.

———— �֍ ————

Helen was the fourth daughter, she was my mother's mother. She was my grandmother. A non-recovering Catholic. Raised in the church, literally. She was an early emotional incest victim, and co- dependent wrapped in one. She was there for her father at all times. She became the surrogate "pastor's wife" when Father John's wife, her mother, died suddenly when the kids were in their early teens. Helen became his emotionally incestual substitute wife! She scrubbed floors in the parish, cleaned the vestments, bought the wine, cooked for the parish pot lucks and for her sisters and dad.

She had been the "religiously correct", i.e., Catholic guilt daughter, who couldn't go the show biz route because she felt that was too risque. She had no use for her sisters "drinkin', smokin' and screwin" as she quietly and politely would share at times. She knew that God would send them directly to Hell, "do not pass go, do not collect $200, just straight to hell", or worse - to Purgatory. Catholics know what that means! So she was gonna be good, extra good.

So my eventual grandmother, in own her mind, a totally respectful Catholic, got married early and was gonna have a baby, a good Catholic baby in a good blessed Catholic marriage. And live happily ever after.

Well, surprise Helen. One day she came home, pregnant and all, and found hubby was outta there! He must have read some Horace Greely books, so he headed West, young man! Far west, they had lived on the Atlantic Shore, so he moved to Long Beach, California on the Pacific Shore.

She was left to bring the kid, my mother Marian, into the world on her own. So, it was time to move back in with dad in the parish and take up the duties again as surrogate pastor's wife. Obedient and reverent. Since Marian, my mother, was born in the 'teens, as in 1918, it was an era when divorces were not okay, single parents were a total No-No. As her mother was scrubbing those church floors, Marian would hear her mother whine, "If only men weren't such pigs, I wouldn't have gotten pregnant, I wouldn't be burdened with you, and I wouldn't be here living in the church with my father and I'd be happy." Not the most nurturing stuff for Marian to hear, nor a good thing for her feelings about men later in her life!!

In the meantime, as little Marian grew up she wanted to meet her birth father. Her mom, Helen, never remarried they just lived in the church with Father John. Her father had had no contact with his wife Helen once he left her, except to send child support checks to her a number of times a year. Marian traced him down through those payments, and started writing him when she was about 10. Since she had no real contact with him and he was 3000 miles away in Southern California, in her mind, he had become the absent "golden knight" type of a dad. Part of a syndrome that happens with kids whose father abandons them. They build this picture of this awesome, loving man who they know is somewhere just thinking of them all the time and that things would be PERFECT in her life, if... if she could just be with him. He would never spank her, yell at her, never refuse to give her money to buy what she wanted, nor make her do chores... like her ogre mother was doing. He would be loving, giving, perfect.

She saved up and when she was 18, she got a relative to go with her on the Greyhound bus to California to see her perfect father.

When she got to his house in Long Beach, she went up to the door and knocked. His wife opened the door, Marian told her she wanted to see "Mr. Miller", it was important, and that he was expecting her. He came to the door. Marian said "Hello father, I'm your daughter, Marian." He yelled at her, to get away, to never bother him again, to stop the insane letters and Christmas cards. That in his mind - she was dead. Very dead.

He slammed the door in her face. She was broken. This was NOT the dream fantasy she had had of them meeting, him hugging her, telling her how special she was... Nope. Any wonder then why she had men issues later in life??

———— ✴ ————

Young Marian, my mother, then returned to New Jersey. She went to work. She wanted to become a "star" like her aunts. She turned to dancing with a vengeance. Rejected by her father, living with a disturbed and disturbing mother. She made it to the auditions for the famous Radio City Music Hall Rockette's. She was ready to become a Rockette, when her mother pulled the guilt trip on her, beat her down about religion, inappropriateness of behavior of show biz and what tramps her aunts all were, and that God was not pleased with her aunts...

So Marian gave up the show biz thing and turned to become a "respectable working girl" as a secretary. This was something respectable and expected for a woman to be in that era, particularly a woman whose mother and father had been divorced! Shame, shame.

A side note, when I grew up, even though our family was only average income, and we lived in a regular post World War II WASP suburb, I was told by my mother to never play with kids who came from divorced homes, or who lived in apartments, since they were not good enough! We knew what 'those people' were like. A throwback to her childhood issues!

In time, Marian became a bitter, unhappy, suppressed secretary. A person who never got ulcers, but gave everyone else ulcers! NEVER owning her own anger but she expressed her anger through others. She had been hurt as a child, both by her mother and her father. She had issues with men as well as women. So, she eventually had to have a child of her own, so she could "have something to love and that would love her forever!" REMEMBER those words, sadly over the years as a teacher, counselor and therapist, I've heard a version of those words so often from young ladies, from their teen years on up, when I would be talking the "be careful dating, you could get pregnant mini-lecture" I had so many say that line. Sad for the girl and would be sad for the baby.

Those words by Marian were the unhealthy beginning of a smothering, destructive, possessive mother. And a living Hell for me being that baby.

Hmmm, I must have known what lay ahead as I lay in her womb! I didn't want to come out into the world and face the music. Marian who was only 4'11"and 97 pounds and was carrying this (me) 8½ pound baby boy. The delivery was horrendous. She was in labor for days even after a legendary quick car trip with her brother-in-law Sam over a cobblestone and trolley tracked street in downtown Bloomfield, New Jersey, where he hoped to induce the labor! I was due on the 5th of August, but that dragged on until the 20th! I was fighting reality all the way already! The hospital was in a major city, Newark, New Jersey, but it was a strict traditional catholic hospital, no "C" sections, because it was against God's will!

So, after days of protracted labor, I was finally born. Both of my eyes were black and blue, my right eye remained shut and puffed for weeks, my left eye stayed shut for a long time. My head was slightly "tweaked" by the forceps used to try to yank this puppy outta momma. I looked totally beaten up! And I was.

Due to that difficult delivery, my father and mother were told there was a good chance I would be blind, very possibly mentally retarded and maybe even deaf due to that rough delivery. Good start! So, yup, I prolly already knew what was in store for me. Oh well, at least it got me good stuff for a book on - you guessed it - Emotional Incest, an often ignored topic.

❏ ❏ ❏ ❏

"I Never Got to be a Little Boy"

What was the Fodder for making me be a poster child for ACOA??!!! Well, going back in the story a bit, yes, my mother, Marian, got married. Twice, or was it once but two men? More on that point later. However, thanks to her father issues, her having major issues with men came naturally. As a little girl growing up having heard all those "wonderful" things about men from her mother - as in an -*'all men are pigs'* - sort of way, she had a skewed view of men/marriage/life. Marian had a husband - Jim, Sr. But she really wanted a *'father'* to replace the absent father she had growing up... So her hubby became her father, her baby, Jim Jr., as in me, became her hubby, so "Let the destruction begin..."

As a kid, I had no extended family to speak of. My father, Jim Sr., had a brother, Sam who was married and had one child who was six weeks younger than me. My paternal grandfather was dead before I was born, and of course, my grandfather on my mother's side, as we learned earlier, had said goodbye to the family before mother was even born.

My paternal grandmother was a possessive overbearing controlling bitch on wheels. She ran both of her son's lives into the ground the best she could, and drove her husband to an early death. I never did find out her issues, it was something no one talked about. I just heard and saw, what grandma Gordon had done to my father particularly. And once, when I was only about 5, I had this loving lady (not!!) push me - her damn grand child - off her lap with disdain, saying, "go away, how could you be part of my family. You've got blue eyes, and blond hair. We all have black hair and brown eyes!" Rejection by your grandmother is not good for a kid's self-esteem. Didn't she read "the book" about how much grandmothers are supposed to love their little grandchildren whether they are urchins or Einsteins! Tender she wasn't!

My other grandmother (aka "nanny"), my mother's mom, Helen of the Parscouta sisters (known on stage as Park Sisters), the one who chose to NOT be an heathen in her words and be an actress like the other sisters, was outta the picture pretty much for my childhood too. She was very European in demeanor, but lost in the world. She had continued to make herself even more miserable about her divorce when she was left with little Marian to raise alone. She drove her self hard, and punished herself. She worked hard and ended up with what in those days was termed a nervous breakdown, followed by a 1950's diagnosis of "hardening of the arteries to the brain", today the parallel would be dementia or Alzheimer's. There was no treatment or help nor understanding of aging, as there is today. Eventually she was put into a state mental hospital with other patients who ran the gamut of severely emotionally dysfunctional to the severely intellectually disabled and low functioning. This was a bummer for a smart woman like Helen, who knew pretty much what was going on, but whose memory was failing quickly. Today, it might be just old age, Dementia, or even Alzheimers, but then it meant warehousing in the looney bin - Marlboro State Hospital in New Jersey's farm area! Yes, Jersey has farming, and the infamous large Jersey Beefsteak tomatoes are prime examples.

It was extremely depressing for me as a kid to go with mom to see "nanny Helen" at that state hospital. Guards every where and walled in. Wailing mental cases. Scary folks staring into nothing. Dungeons of doom.

On one summertime visit to see Nanny, I remember going to the hospital with my mom, and as often happened, Nanny was out doing what they called "occupational therapy", i.e., doing manual labor picking those aforementioned Beefsteak Tomatoes in a field. Vegetables picking vegetables in 90° weather. Classic Jersey summer 90% humidity, middle of August as my mother and I waited for Nanny to return from the fields where she had been sent to harvest the tomatoes! We watched as the hospital "labor" bus (excuse me, therapy bus) rolled in mid-afternoon. Nanny and the rest of the confused and mixed up fools - hot, sweaty, dirty, clothes dusty, bandanas and babushka's on their heads, tired and bedraggled, got off the bus to greet their visiting families. *'It was good for them... it was therapy.'* said the staff. Yeah, tell that one to Freud. People who were almost mental vegetables themselves, picking vegetables! Hmmm. A 1950's psychological approach to help.

Then, on another 'wonderful' Marlboro State Hospital visit and childhood experience to visit my Nanny - my mother and I were required to be there to 'witness' Nanna receiving electroconvulsive shock therapy. My mother had to be there since it was a controversial new tool that was to be tried on these old duff's to get their brains to function. Of course the idea was to wipe out the old information in those little grey cells, aiming for the bad info that was messing up their heads but wiping out all, good with the bad. Then the idea was, they would re-train the person with good healthy information. And all would end happy and well again. That was the Theory... but NOT always the reality, trust me.

For whatever wisdom, the state wasn't just satisfied with a release signed by my mother who was legally responsible for her mother, but they required my mother to also be present, albeit in the hallway, but present when the "treatment" was done. The walls were not sound proof. A number of patients were fortunate(??) enough to be 'treated' at the same time. This made for the families waiting in the hallway, a not too pleasant place or experience as they heard their grandmothers and grandfathers do a bit of screaming as the electro-shocks wiped out the bad parts of the brains memory, along with the majority of the good memory. Zombies they call them in movies. Sitting there with my mother, it was not a nice sound for an eight year old to hear, the screams of pain of his grandmother. What a pleasant family outing! What pleasant memories for this kid, with one grandmother saying, "hey you can't be mine, I don't like you" and the other being tortured and abused in the name of medical science. Nanna died lost and confused in the state hospital, after being there for 8 years. An ignominiously sad way to leave this world. She never did have a clue who I was, or what I was doing tagging along with my mother. She'd look at me with total LOSS in her eyes as I'd try to hug her and call her Nanny... Oh well. More to add to the ACA fodder.

Overall, my mother, the possessive twit that she had become with all her bad experiences in life taking their toll, didn't want me to have much to deal with anyone outside the immediate family, i.e., she and I would be all she and I needed, PERIOD! "Love honor and obey, til death do us part." Even Jim, Sr., was persona non gratis. She wanted just herself and her little man, what more did she need now? This meant keeping me away from what little birth family there was, which was just Uncle Sam, his wife Lillian and their son, my only cousin - Bobby.

Later it turns out there were some other options that were not taken advantage of. My paternal grandpa - though he was dead before I was born - did have brothers, and those brothers had families with kids, but my father had nothing to do with them for some reason, and never mentioned them. I didn't find out about his uncle until after my father died and my Aunt Lillian mentioned how neither her husband Sam, nor my father, ever talked about nor reached out to their uncle. I don't know and never will why. But it was in concert with my mother wanting no competition for my love and attention. In fact, she bitched whenever the relative's (Aunt Lil, Uncle Sam and Bobby) were to come visit, or when she, my father and little Jimmy (me!) were invited to visit them up at their home in Northern Jersey, across from NYC. On more than one trip to Aunt Lil's and Uncle Sam's, the ride up ended in a heated argument with my father about the visit, so it would mean turning the car around and heading back home when we were already half way there.

Later, I found out why she would make such disparaging remarks about them, and do her best to keep their contact to a minimum. She had a few secrets!

I was an only child (or was that a lonely child, or both?). I asked about having sisters and brothers over and over. I wanted them, but was told by mother that after the difficult delivery of ME - i.e., it was my Fault (guilt!) - that mother's insides were so torn up she could never have any more children. So, the point was, "get over it Jimmy, there will be no more children, no siblings, and thus, it was my duty to make things right for her, be there for her, etc." Hmm, it's the least I could do after all the damage I caused, right? I owed her my company and companionship. Emotional Incest with full caps.

I wanted "kid" company, and often asked if my cousin could come down from the city to our shore home, or if I could go up there to visit. One of the picture in the book is that cousin and I on the beach which was

45

two doors down the street from our home. I just wanted to be with other kids. I wanted to be a "little boy". Unconsciously, I already knew I was the "little man, not the kid". I had been trained indirectly into what it took to be a little man and what my responsibilities were. I wasn't allowed to have kid visitors, because, according to mother, most kids were evil, including my cousin Bobby who was one of the most evil according to her. Whenever any kids visited, after they left, I got a long "martyr" dissertation from my mother, about how much trouble their visit and presence had been, how horrible they all were - they ate too much, made messes for her, etc. Her point was - why would I want other kids around, when I could have fun with her(i.e. why would I reject her when she had done so much for me, including almost die due to my difficult 5 hour birth!) After all, I... we, were all each other needed... Guilt for days and accompanied by pointing out how "bad" the visiting kids were for me, that they were bad bad bad influences whether the visit was for a few hours or those horrible times for her, the 3 or 4 times in my life, I was allowed to have a kid friend "sleep over". The beginning of a modified Munchausen Syndrome as we'll see later also.

This deemed me to a lonely isolated childhood. My options I was offered were basically - mother, or no one.

In the 1990's, while sitting around with my life partner Ross one day, we were comparing our mother issues. One of the reasons we hit it off originally was that we both had distanced ourselves from our mothers, something normally is seen negatively but for our relationship, it was a positive beacon that we had something in common! That day, as we talked, I brought up my mother wanting me home a lot as a kid. I remembered staying home, being absent, from school a whole lot. Ross' experience was the opposite, he had years and years of perfect attendance.

He was in disbelief that any parent would NOT want their kid to be in school! So, out came my old reports cards to show him the proof. I have all my old report cards from first grade on, yeah I'm OCD on some things. I had skipped kindergarten, so just first grade on. On each report card, for each year, the days absent - 68, 70, 65, 84... Considering that the average school year was a total of 170 school days, I missed almost half of the school days each damn year! Mother would come in to my bedroom and say, "Jimmy, its raining and dreary, why don't you just go back to sleep, stay in and later you and I can go out for a nice lunch together, just you and I." Or, "It's Monday, its cold, stay in today, take a long weekend, you deserve it. You look tired". Or, "You've missed Monday and Tuesday this week, why don't I just write a note for you to school, and you stay home the rest of the week so you can start fresh on Monday and we'll run into NYC to the Bronx Zoo?" Many week long absences, and quite a few for two weeks!

And what happened if little Jimmy was stupid enough to reject the offer and went to school against

Mother's so-called wishes and concerns? Well, let me tell you one classic example. On the east coast, in New Jersey, where I attended elementary school, and junior high, the schools were big old brick things, with classic indoor hallways that all had a traditional school building smell of books, mopped floors and lunches in the kid's lockers. One of my 8th grade experiences of going to school against mothers wishes, was the most scary and vivid in my memory so I'll share.

Remember, I was just that, "Little Jimmy", I was smaller and younger than my classmates because I had started school early, I was enrolled in 1st grade when I was just 4 yrs and 11 months old, and started classes the week I turned 5 in the first grade. So I was the youngest in my grade each year, at least 6 months and usually a year or more younger than the rest of the students each year - plus I was not a big dude. As an adult I'm only 5'8", so as a kid, I was just a little guy.

Oh well, back to this 8th grade scenario that I mentioned in Part One. I was struggling with lots of personal and family issues at that point, and here I was sitting in Mr. Ryder's 4th period Social Studies Class. It was just before lunch, and at one point, Mr. Ryder looked at Jimmy and said, "well, Mr. Jimmy, guess what...? here comes your mother down the hallway... again. Take your books and I guess you'll be going home... again...!" He always said it with a special sneer and twinge of hostility. And sure enough, down the hallway for all the effen world to see would come my screwed up mother, a true vision of loveliness, this time in a bathrobe! Often with the bathrobe not completely buttoned up, earing nothing, her tits hangin' out, having had a drink,... or twenty that morning and/ or maybe a few Miltowns or Equanil's, the prescription tranquilizer of choice at that time. Then, off would go Jimmy and mom, down the school hallway, heading home to an afternoon of "togetherness". She had rescued little Jimmy once again from those terrible people and the evil kids.

We would be together and share the rest of the day, and prolly the rest of the week, because now I'd be too embarrassed to go back to school too soon. The catcalls from the other kids about Mother - floppy boobs and all - showing up in her bathrobe were not such a positive thing for me, or for my self esteem. Little did I realize that I was also struggling not only with being the "best little boy", but struggling with being a little faggot too! No, not the nellie queen type. I was always into cars and trucks, and even had my own real full sized car in the back yard to work on, play with, and make believe I was driving that was left by an old neighbor, from the time I was five years old! But I was definitely different from many of the other boys and not into sports, though I certainly seemed to like girls for dancing and fun at the time. I was confused for sure.

Often the damn teachers got on the bandwagon too, making snide and cruel remarks about my mother and I, many times in front of the rest of the students. I remember Mrs. Newman, my algebra teacher, bringing me to tears when I was in the 8th grade. I was in section 8A White, which is what my group was called, it was an intermediate school - 7th and 8th grades only, and the grades were divided up into A, B and C groups. In those days, it was still politically correct to put the "smart kids" nowadays referred to as "gifted" in the A group, the "average kids" in the B group, and the "blue collar", gonna be laborer type dumbbells in the C group. Weirdly, some of my best friends were the ones in the C group, I was impressed that they seemed to have less school work and easier times than I and be happier! And they were cool kids. But here I was in front of Mrs. Newman's class, I had just come back from a two week absence due to illness (more mental illness, then physical, another case of 'alcoholic motherism'!!!) That day I couldn't do one of the algebra problems at the board because I had missed the lesson during the last few weeks covering the topic - well, Mrs. Newman made a point of informing OUTLOUD all the kids in class that I was an example of what would happen if "you stayed home with you mother and ignored your schooling duties, like Jimmy does".

Classic drizzly school day as a kid, and this is what I got from Mother: "It's a dreary day, why don't you stay home?" or "It's cold out, sleep in and I'll write you a note that I overslept and didn't get you to school on time." or "Stay home today, and we can go to Dennis's restaurant in Red Bank for lunch." Or "It's already Wednesday, so why don't you stay home the rest of the week, and go back on Monday?" or "I know you didn't get your school project finished, so why don't you stay home today and work on it, I'll write you a note." Oh my.

Like Hell bitch! Was it my choice to be 'married' to her??? My mother was the so-called adult here, my so called parent and mother and was to be teaching me what was right and wrong. Not instead what was sick and sicker! Listening to Mrs. Newman, I got so embarrassed I had to go to the nurses office to throw up! Then, guess what, mother got to come to school and once again rescue her little boy and take me home. Such a damn mixed message, reinforcing the wrong sick things. And as we'll see in a bit, where was Dad when I had to go home and be spouse to Mom?

❑ ❑ ❑ ❑

Dad, oh where, oh where is Dad?

ACOA issues? Parent drinking issues? Father issues? Emotional Incest issues? Everyone has issues as a kid? Damn, maybe I did have a semi- normal childhood? Are you connecting with any of your own issues? Or friends issues? Often folks read books like this thinking it's about "those people" only to find, "damn some of this is about me too". Remember, it's what we learn AFTER we know every thing that helps! So where the hell was my dad? And an FYI here, I never called or knew my father as "dad" but from the time I was 5, I called him Jim. I was trying to ask him something, and saying 'dad' didn't work, so I did like my mother, and yelled, JIM! And he listened so forever he was Jim to me... He was working extra hours to 'save the family'. Yeah sure. Save his own ass maybe! In the state of New Jersey, there were "blue laws" in those days of my youth, North Jersey still has them - which meant - no business allowed to be open on Sunday other than food and dining. And also, very few stores were open during the week at night in those days. You shopped during the day before 6. Friday and Thursday nights is when many stores did stay open late. But Big Jim, as in my father, in his infinite wisdom and quest for failure, being the gifted, pissed, misguided misanthrope that he was, decided to open a hobby store and be open every evening Monday through Friday til 9 pm, so he could go there directly from his blue collar work at a Jersey Shore military base. AND then be open Saturday and Sunday 10 am til 9 pm! He said it was to make money and help make financial ends meet. He was working at the time for the Federal Government, having failed at getting his own business rolling. So this part time gig of having a hobby store (model trains, model cars and model airplanes) was an EXCUSE to allow him to stay away from the home as much as possible. Gave him a somewhat legitimate excuse to be distant from the family as in my mother and me! I call it "Busyism" - stay busy so you can't deal with what needs to be dealt with. Over the years as a shrink, I've seen many patients who use Busyism as a way to avoid someone they are married to, or avoid family responsibilities or just hide of Reality.

Big Jim, a mensa candidate, an angry bitter man whose life had been controlled and directed by his possessive smothering 4' 11", 98 pound mother. Does this physical description sound familiar? It is off a pound or two but close enough to, yup, you guessed it from Marian, my mother. Well, from a psychological perspective, he married his mother - damn - Freud had some good stuff about this and was right on! Ironically, Big Jim, who waited until he was 40 to marry, even brought home my mother, his wife (mother replacement?) to live at home with his mother for a year or so when they got married. Was this an unofficial power issue, was this "the changing of the guard"? My first year out of the womb was spent with mother, father and little Jimmy living with Grandma Gordon.

She's the one I pointed out earlier who pushed me off her knee when I was five years old saying I wasn't a real Gordon. She did NOT like my mother. Grandma was a social climber and wanted my father to marry into money, into society not marry a 'hussy' (a woman or girl who's attractive but disrespectful or immoral) who was a former stage dance, now a lowly secretary in an office. Grandma hated Marian so it was a way of Jim getting back at his mother for his childhood issues. Damn Freud scores again.

As a kid, I remember my father pointing out old cars as we would drive around, "see that old Ford there, I had one, I wrapped it around a telephone pole one night when I was drunk", or "see that old Hudson there, I had one just like that, I wrecked it one night when I was...drunk" Pattern here? Yup, ACOA fodder to the max. Most old guys point out with a twinge of nostalgia "that old car" that they had loved, or had their first sex in, or raced on the streets - but with Big Jim, it was usually the one he wiped out, after a drink or twenty. Hmmm, was he drinking to avoid Mom? And home? And his life in general? Did he replace heavy drinking with "Busyism"? YUP, you guessed.

Big Jim had the brains. He wanted to follow in his dad's footsteps and be an Builder or Architect. His father had been involved in the building of the Empire State Building and the Hoover Dam. Jim wanted to explore the world, work on projects in Africa, South America, exotic places like his father had been doing and would talk about to Jim. And of course, these were places far from his mother! His dad already was informally teaching Jim, keep busy with jobs that are a 100 miles from home or even better thousands of miles from home so you can avoid responsibilities to the family!

Instead of getting to go into architecture, using his talent in design and engineering, he worked the banker jobs, and resentfully did what his mother wanted for him. Safe local jobs with prestige. For her it was all about social climbing and prestige. He worked in a number of financial institutions "in the city" as in NYC, so Grandma Gordon could tell her friends he was doing big time stuff. Hell, telling them he worked in New York City was much more prestigious than saying he was a teller at a bank in White Haven, PA where she was raised. Part of his resistance routine to passively get back at his mother, was getting fired from a few NYC financial institutions for being quarrelsome and even for telling off customers or other employees. I still have a few letters from Chase Brass where my father was informed he would have to leave if his attitude didn't improve, but it includes the reminder that he was a brilliant man who they would like to keep so "please Jim try to control your temper and help our company grow".

His banking career to satisfy his Mom got sidetracked much to Grandma Gordon's dismay, when Jim got to be one of the last guys drafted, and one of the oldest into World War II. Bitter at being drafted, bitter at still not getting to do his architecture dream,

very anti-President Roosevelt's politics, he went off
to Africa as a US Army airplane mechanic. In a way, it
served a purpose cuz his mother was pissed as crap
that he was a grease- monkey on airplanes instead
of working in administration. For Jim, it was quite a
change in jobs, and scenery that turned out a great
learning experience for him and for Grandma Gordon,
a complete pisser yet passively for Jim, a great way to
get back at his mother.

Turned out, he enjoyed his stay in Africa. He was
actually away from the battlefield and fighting of the
war, instead based at a location where the planes were
brought for repair and servicing. He even had cheap
servant help from the natives. He worked his way up
and down to master Sargent. His anger and temper
interfered again with his success as he told off a few
superiors, then wham, he was demoted again but
would work back up to Sarge. As I found out from my
Aunt Lil later in my life, toward the end of the War while
he was stationed with his Army Squad in the Belgian
Congo area of Africa and on an island at times (don't
hold me to exact geography during that time, since
Jim seldom talked to me at all about his War exploits,
other than a few times pointing out that the two leather
wrapped wine bottles, or a few coins he had amongst
his stuff came from his days in the Belgian Congo but
with no details) that he wrote his Brother, as in Aunt
Lil's husband, and later my Uncle Samuel, "You won't
be hearing from me or be able to contact me for a
while, probably many months, as I'm being sent to

Ascension Island on a project". And classic Jim, he never mentioned that to me, or my mother while I was growing up. I had to learn it from Aunt Lil and she only knew it was a special military project. The War ended a few months later. Much of the Military Air Support for the fighting in Europe was based in parts of Africa so since he was a mentally gifted guy, who knows why he was sent to the island on a Secret Mission.

When World War 2 ended, he reluctantly returned to the states. That is one thing he did share with me and everyone when I was a kid, that he always wished he could return to the Republic of Congo in Africa forever and never have to be in the US again. Shortly after arriving back home, he met my future mother Marian, just before he was to be discharged. She was about 13 years younger than he was. She was a lively active person, had a good dancer body, and in good shape. He was already "old", handsome and debonaire looking, quiet and but moody. He was still angry at the world for not giving him, or letting him get what he wanted out of LIFE. Bitter. He liked to read and do quiet things, while she liked to be active and outgoing. But, unconsciously she was looking for that father she hadn't had as mentioned earlier in this book. And he was looking to replace his controlling mother, so someone could continue to "whip" him emotionally and give him an excuse for his failures. Welcome to Marian, his future wife, my soon to be mother. What a mismatch in some ways, but a good score in others so he could remain angry, beaten, and have a good reason to...DRINK and drink somemore!

So my Dad was not really interested in being a father, not really interested in being a husband, as mentioned he married my mother mostly to ANNOY his mother! Yeah, they loved each other enough to live together til 'death did them partt' 40+ years. Mostly he was just interested in being an angry curmudgeon about the misery of living. Growing up I remember mostly every morning, coming out to find my father sitting at the kitchen counter, drinking his coffee, with his head in his hands grumbling about how miserable life was. He would pound his forehead with his wrist as he bitched about everything from the family not getting up early enough, to having car payments (who doesn't), to the political climate. Always something. Never a happy man. And the grass was always greener somewhere OTHER than were he was. Africa, Samoa, South America, at any outpost the government had jobs where he "knew life was better than wherever" he was.

He worked as a blue collar worker after the war until he retired at 70 from Federal Government as a Civil Servant. Never able to hold his temper, he could not become management so suffered doing regular hands-on work instead of a desk job. And this was not unlike his younger years when his mother would get him his jobs through her social connections, since he was her favorite son, and she so wanted him to be a bank president and success, that now his wife, surrogate mother, Marian, who worked on the same Military base, and later in personnel departments (now called HR) was the one who kept his job for him when he would mess up with anger and tell bosses off. When we moved to California, I remember over hearing a discussion with my mother and her boss, she was now working for the personnel department on the Army base, he said that Jim, Sr. needed to be careful or he would get let go, but the director liked my mother Marian, so they worked it out for him to keep his job. Without her presence, he would have had to hit the streets many times.

In a sense, I feel that the blue collar work he did was a direct slap, a passive aggressive behavior, at his mother who envisioned the white collar successful executive son she wanted so badly. I think he revelled in working greasy dirty jobs, driving a truck and never having a tie and white shirt on, as a way of telling his mother to fuck off.

Later when the store failed, and the family moved to California, he 'conveniently' got a job assignment off the coast on an island. The military base, Pt. Mugu Naval Air Staion, had tracking stations on the islands off the coast of California. He would fly out Monday morning and return late Friday. The weekend then could be 'lost' with a few drinks, and in getting prepared to go back to work on Monday. Laundry, shopping, etc. And it also allowed him the opportunity to claim NO responsibility at home for anything from needed home repairs to buying cars to my school affairs since he could play "martyr" and remind how he was out of the loop by being gone so much, "so what does my opinion mean anyway? You two seem to make all the plans and decisions." His favorite way out of making decisions. Hmmm, again forcing a spousal relationship between myself and my mother, as we made all the household decisions from buying cars to choice of carpet to even decisions regarding the limited contact with his own damn mother. Usually the decisions were mine, and my mother normally went along with her emotionally married husband - ME - and whatever choices I made. I had Power at 11, 14, 18, whatever. Without realizing it, I had power and while, I was never a "classic little boy", nor having the kid fun kids are supposed to have, it was kinda cool to be in control of things. And, yes, still today, I am not good to this day at NOT having some control of things whether at home, work, associations I belong to, or just Life.

In fact, it took me until I was 40 years old to be able to fly in an airplane cross country and be able to 'give over' that power to the pilot! Though, I also realize, I had been looking for some healthy parenting for years and once I trusted a doctor, masseuse, even a friend, I did really like to sit back and let them do their work. To put myself under their control. A version of allowing them to take care of the "Little Jimmy" inside of me. To this day, I have many friends who I appreciate because I trust them to take care of me. As I mention from time to time in this book, it is never to late for a happy childhood with healthy parenting even when those parents might be decades younger than you!

———— ➤✺◄ ————

So dad, Jim Sr., was not very 'there' for the family, physically there but emotionally there? As a parent there? NOPE. For instance, when Marian was doing her most intense prescription drug abuse (those infamous Miltowns/Meprobamate) plus her controlling drinking shtick, I was in Junior High/Intermediate School. At that time, Big Jim avoided reality with a passion. Claiming that he needed to be at his hobby store 24/7, 365 days a year to make money to save the family. He never closed the store except for Christmas Day in the afternoon, and even then he would just come home a few hours early! Is there an avoidance issue here?

Yup, even for Thanksgiving dinners, when it was the one day a year where it was Jim's turn to have his mother down for the day versus the norm when Grandma Gordon would go to Uncle Sam's for holidays, birthdays etc with the excuse that Uncle Sam lived only a half hour away from her vs our home being an hour and half away, it was my mother and I who would go pick her up, NOT Jim. Mother and I would drive up, bring her down and get stuck entertaining her while Jim, Sr. stayed at his store until the last minute even on Thanksgiving. So, since Uncle Sam and Aunt Lil lived close to Grandma, they got her most of the time, but we got her Thanksgiving Day. What a turkey she was!

And she would grumble and gripe but never taking it out on her favorite son, Jim. My mother and I got all the negative vibes while she would justify how wonderful her favorite son Jim was that he was working so hard for all of us. Even though it was obvious to her other son Sam, and anyone who saw the actions that Jim was... REJECTING his mother.

Passive aggressively, never telling her what he really thought of her, but just avoiding her physically and emotionally. I NEVER saw them hug! Let alone have her give him a good bye kiss on the cheek when visits were over. But she favored him. Ironically, sadly, Uncle Sam died when I was 12, and we still lived in New Jersey. We moved West the next year. That was the basic end of contact with Grandma Gordon for my father. So for the rest of her years, Aunt Lil, Sam's wife, got stuck taking care of Grandma Gordon in her 80's, Grandma Gordon was stuck having her least favorite son's wife 'be there' for her as she slowly aged into a Senior Home from her apartment, with some hospital visits and eventually died. Aunt Lil oversaw it all, even to the funeral and her burial. While her favorite son, Jim, had even gone further away than California, he went to GUAM in the Pacific to work on a government contract for 2 years. That way he got away from his mother, his wife and his son, yeah that would be me!

The Navy civil service contract he was on, offered him the opportunity at no cost 2 round trip flights a year to come home from GUAM but he chose not to take them but instead went to visit Japan instead. AND when Grandma Gordon got very sick in New Jersey, and was expected to die, I wrote and reminded him (as the good parent that I was) that the government would fly him all the way back to New Jersey to be with her during her last days. 16,000 mile round trip for no cost, but NOPE his response to me was, "There isn't really anything I can do for her now anyway."

Well back to my whining about things with my mother, when her drinking and drug episode got majorly out of hand, it was Me - little Jimmy - at 11 to 13 years old, who had to trace down the many doctors that mother was using to get her prescriptions from, call those and confront them with the reality and tell them to stop giving her drugs randomly. Creepily they listened to the 11 year old Junior High kid!

Then, I had to track down, and call and cancel the pharmacy prescriptions. I had to contact the liquor stores where she had accounts and beg them not to send anymore booze 'on account'. In those days we didn't have credit cards, but you'd set up an account at the liquor stores, pharmacies that you'd pay off monthly with cash or a check. Next, I would search the house for hidden bottles of booze and pills. Then I get to toss stoned or drunk, mother into the shower to clean her up after she would go days on a binge, get dirty and smelly and ignore her needs and mine - forget my fathers, he met his needs on his own! One of my fav memories (NOT!) was when she would stay in her room, in the winter when it was cold, sometimes snowy, in New Jersey, under her electric blanket, bombed off her gourd. Then she would turn the heat way down in the house in the middle of winter because she was hot, warmed from within by alcohol. I would sit by the forced heater ducts with my shirt spread over the opening to catch the heat when it came on as I was freezing my ass off.

At that point, Marian didn't see the classic drunk's pink elephants they are supposed to see, but instead did smell "phantom gas leaks" and call the gas company, or the fire department to report potential explosions, sometimes a couple of times a week. A number of times the gas guys would take me aside and lecture me (at 11 or 12 years of age) about getting her to not bother them anymore! Just the same as the fire department guys complained to me when she would call them if the gas company wouldn't respond and come out for her phantom explosive gas leak. Like it was my fucking problem to take care of her, hmmm, was I not the kid? Nope, guess not. Did they ever call my father? No, just talked to me - Adult Child of Alcoholic Jimmy!

And guess what? Yes, finally our house did eventually catch fire but not from the damn ass phantom gas leaks my bitch mother had smelled so many times! Instead it was an electrical short that burned out most of the middle of our ranch style house. Fortunately it was one of the times I actually was in school, because the fire started in the ceiling over my bedroom, and the ceiling fell on my bed and burned and melted my foam rubber mattress. My goldfish boiled, and my room was destroyed. Great sight to come home to. Wonderful fond childhood memories. Mother standing there crying about how could this happen to us, even though it mainly my room totally destroyed. Oh yeah, it was inferred by dear mother, with appropriate guilt laid on me, as she was driving me home from school that day when the fire happened, that HAD I been home from school that day as she had asked me to, the fire would possibly have been discovered, that is, assuming I wasn't dead from the burning ceiling falling on my bed if I had 'slept in'.

Later, as an adult in therapy, I was to really realize how pissed I was at my father for avoiding responsibility and leaving 'the marriage relationship duties' to me, but not until after I had smashed many doors with my fists, lost my temper a few too many times, tossed a few kids across the floor when I was teaching, and gotten an ulcer. It was a lot later, in fact, it was a few days after my father died that it hit me - and I realized I got cheated out of being a little boy as much by him, as by my mother. AND THAT'S WHEN I REALIZED where the

ANGER in the alternative book title came from... Life Liberty and the Pursuit of Anger!

❑ ❑ ❑ ❑

Now issues. Today, my office is in Beverly Hills, California 90212 - the 'understated' zip code of BH vs the well known 90210! Hmm, on Beverly Drive, a good address, good karma right? Remember, "If you want to SOAR with the EAGLES... don't hang with the turkeys..."

In my BH office, my patients and clients are attorneys, business folks, wanna be actors and writers, sports figures as well as the real "working" actors who you do see on the television, Netflix or at the movies, and often as not, folks you'll see waiting on your table at a nearby restaurant in between acting jobs!!

My office is located on the second floor of a non-descript understated 1940's brick building which used to house one of the major talent agencies until the 70's when they moved to a new high rise around the corner. Fittingly, the building was originally built by a go-no-where actress who had a very successful early Hollywood director father. He made epics, and became a legend, daughter wanted to be a star, but she became a landlord instead. She eventually opened a celebrity restaurant in the building where the gimmick was naming entree's after its celebrity diners.

This way you could order a "jerry lewis", a 'ham' sandwich on coarse grain rye, or a "jane mansfield", two eggs - yolk up, firm not runny. The "rock hudson", a half chicken dish that you could have 'either way' - broiled or baked. The "judy garland", an appetizer(?) plate of 'fried... vegetables'! Any time of the day or night, there was at least a small crowd in there. Connie specialized in putting plaques on tables honoring regular customers, so they liked sitting at "their" table, under their name "in lights". Not Broadway at Sardi's but South Beverly Drive at Parker's, but then who's counting? I started visiting there with an actress friend of mine, then the 'local legend in her own mind' Angylene who was a kick to hang out with. And I too ended up with a small table top that was decorated with the image of my business card. Fun, silly but a kick for my ego any way.

Today, this building houses shrinks, mid- eastern financial companies, an upstart wanna be talent agency or two, a well known Producer who did the original Willy Wonka, Mel who was a great friend... Yeah, even in Beverly Hills it had a leaky roof plus the often overflowing urinal, and that occasional homeless dude who slips in for a nap, after a few too many nips of booze. Gotta give him credit for knowing how to be a bum with class, or at least a classy address. Interesting place for me.

The street is busy with locals who know that the power players eat and drink here, as well as have their agents, attorneys, dentists, and wax ladies here - wax the eyebrows at Janette's, while sipping your double de-caf frap from Starbucks. Janette probably just came in from a set in a nearby studio (Sony Pix, 20th Century Fox, Paramount, Warner are all a short hop by car from here) where she did the make-up for one of her many celeb clients who will have only Janette do their make-up.

Tourists stick to Rodeo Drive which is a block away, and filled with tourists. If only the tourists knew where to really spot stars then the privacy here on Beverly Drive or on Canon would be gone, one of the best kept secrets in LA.

For 10 years I had an annex office in Hollywood, yes, the famous Hollywood. My office was on a seedy side street over looking a female mud wrestling emporium. What an appropriate locale for my office running court ordered Domestic Violence Batterers groups for men who abuse their wives, girlfriends and lovers? Very much unlike the glorious pretentious perception the average tourist has about Hollywood. The Hollywood office gets the lower caste of our society. seedy, dirty, losers. One of the wife beater clients there came in dirty every time after rummaging through trash dumpsters to retrieve enough aluminum cans to redeem so he has enough money for his class.

Did you ever hear of Needles, California? While sorting myself out and figuring who I really was, I ended up taking on a part time staff position at a community hospital there. I was working primarily in the small stroke rehab unit. Two times a month I made the trek across 300 miles of arid desert to this "garden spot" on the Colorado River! Home of cactus, mesquite scrub brush, scorpions and the occasional gila monster that wanders over from the Arizona side.

The hospital is in a "rural needs" area as defined by federal and state codes. That means in shorthand - desperate conditions. The true definition is "a location that is more than 30 miles or 30 minutes of driving time from the center of a metropolis of a 150,000 people or more..." It was established originally along a major railroad route for safety of crews. Then as the Interstate Highway system took over the country in the 1950's and 60's, there needed to be hospitals for accidents and other emergency situations along the interstate routes. Thus that small 20 bed hospital got to stay alive with special funding over the years. Kewl place for me to be on staff as a "doctor" even though I was a Ph.D., not medical doc of course, but I played a good role with the Rehab/Stroke unit.

Excellent growing time as I realized more about myself than I had ever expected. I got to talk with some great old folks who would be Snow Birds, coming to the town from the cold north, or Canadian towns. Since they were retired folks, they often had health issues including mostly strokes that strike seniors, and dementia/Alzheimer's. I always say that it is when we lose a life of a friend or relative, or our own lives get challenged by health issues, that we really start to totally appreciate our health and well being. Is is a time to reflect on what LIFE is about, and I certainly got to do that there with my stroke patients. I learned so much, so very much. And it was honest and awesome to have medical staff, patients, families compliment my abilities. To get that phone call in LA from nurses in Needles asking for advice on how to deal with someone, or asking when was I due back in Needles again since they were having a problem with a patient. Honest, no strings attached compliments!

Something I had not had as a kid, then they were hooks for something else.

Amidst these stints in brick and mortar places during that time of my life, I had a my "mobile office", which was a sheriff's patrol car. I have spent a bit of my time in the community as a member of a Public Safety Commission for West Hollywood, a consultant/ instructor for the Los Angeles Sheriff's Department, and 'hands on' at the local station. I patrol as a Volunteer and for years was teaching community based policing at the Sheriff's Academy. Thus, the black and whites qualify as an office too since a significant amount my time for almost 30 years, was spent rolling the streets of the city, seeing the 'other side of the city, the city at it's worst - raw, no makeup, deranged, angry, defensive, scared, hurt, in pain, shot up, dead and sometimes at its best, when paramedics save a life, a deputy talks a family into staying together, neighbors respond to help a neighboring family after a fire, along with hearing some very human stories from the deputies as they drive 'their' streets in search of helping humanity. I have stepped aside to just be helping with administrative duties with only an occasional patrol night.

Post the Rodney King riots, I was consulting with the commission that was investigating the Sheriff's relationship with the black community, and the rest of the populus. Here is a little tidbit from the Kolt's Commission referring to the committee that I was on with the GLSCC where our team of five, got commended for our work and the Commission, in it's 500 page plus report, took four pages to recommend the work our committee had done be used as the "template for the entire LA Sheriff Department". Our recommendations included things like, "on patrol, keep the front windows open unless severe rain, so the community members can feel more connection with the deputies" vs cites where they have the windows up 24/7, 365 days a year keeping the connection at a minimum. Nice gentle pat on the back that came from folks I respected by that time, better than my mothers superfluous words that were meant to win me over for her benefit.

❑ ❑ ❑ ❑

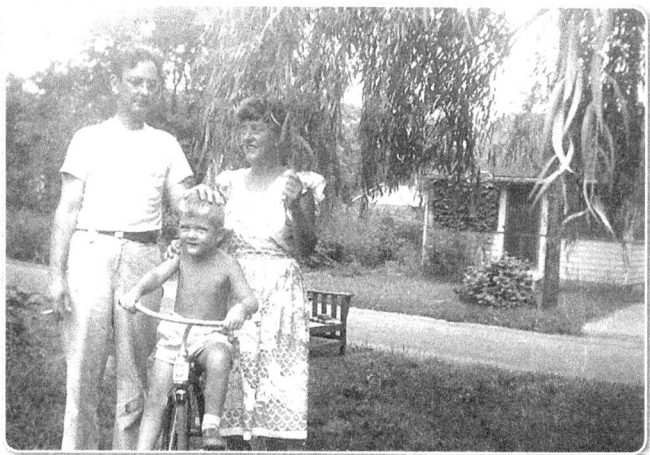

Emotional incest in others lives: Peer counselor Mark's life has been around the big hitters in the entertainment industry. When Mark speaks it is in publicist/hollywood jargon; there never is a simple "hi how are you", but everything is always phrased in superlatives and puffery. One time when he subbed and led my group when I was on the East Coast, when I called after group to see how it went, if there were any problems, and was looking for, "Group went well, everyone participated". Instead I got, "Hello the magnificent Dr. G, yes, your top rated peer counselor Mark, led the group of rich narcissistic miscreants of society with amazing aplomb."

Mark is great at writing and constructing reality but has problems it. He has, and has had, major issues with the women he dates or marries, and there have been plenty of both - the issues and women! He pontificates that all women marry men to emasculate then and they are out to get you. Ah, but I challenged him that he loved his mother, who only recently at 94 expired. And, duh, she was a woman! For his whole life, they were in daily contact, emails, phone, visits, etc. She had apartment downstairs from his penthouse in Beverly Hills. So maybe(?) Mom, was the one who really emasculated him, who he is mad at, but instead of being a "bad son", has "transferred" the issues that he himself should deal with, onto the gals he dates.

His Dad had divorced Mom early in Mark's life and Mom reminded him often how lucky she was to have Mark to fill in the gaps left in her life first due to the divorce then to the early death of her ex.

Mark would never admit to being in an emotional incest situation because there was no sexual pairing. That made him feel safe but damn, as with others I will prolly mention, gals realized when they started dating Mark, they got two for one! And got Mom too!!!

My French friend, Pierre, is another where when you date him, or even just become friends, you get "Mum too". Thirty six years old, a peer counselor and PR person. He was an actor in high school and had two friends he did plays with commit suicide. He was devastated and still does suicide hotline hours. At this point, he still living with mom 80% of the time. Yes, he has his own place 10 minutes from Mum's for the last few years. He and Mum both have nice places by the coast also, separate but even there, just walking distance from each other. His mother and father split up then divorced before he was born. Dad has supported Pierre and his mum plus mom inherited some condominiums that she started renting out many years ago.

Pierre travels constantly working for an airline, so since Mum's place is on the way to the airport AND she does his laundry, cooks for him and he has never moved full time into his own place. He doesn't know how to cook or do laundry so Mum is happy to her 'guy' there all the time. And, wow when you have dinner with them, whether at home or dining out, they bicker and bicker all the way through the meal, yes like an old married couple. They will look at your from time to time with the facial expression, "can you believe what he is saying?" and he will whisper sometimes, "she never stops!".

❑ ❑ ❑ ❑

Life Liberty and the Pursuit of ANGER

As I work on this book, more and more, I realize that my story is and was the Life, Liberty and Pursuit of ANGER that I kid about, and was naming the book originally. Why? As an aside, its amazing how the anger builds and comes out in other ways. Here is one of my examples of acting out, that could have caused much grief and could have been very disastrous. In the early 1980's when I had my own tour bus company, taking folks around the west coast and to places like Vegas and to ski lodges, as a way to pay for my grad studies, I had one big episode that was especially memorable and I traced back to internal childhood anger. Yeah, that sounds like something a therapist would say, so remember I am a therapist and many in my field, unconsciously, DO go into it to work out our issues.

My bus was a real bus, a former greyhound cross country bus, 40 feet long, 13 feet high, and weighing about 55,000 pounds with capacity of 50 folks. A real bus, you've seen the old Greyhounds in movies with an upstairs and downstairs, not the little things on van chassis. Being a nerd that I am, I had modified it. I have always loved driving and mechanical things. Most busses in those days had automatic transmissions and were good for 80 mph. Not good enough for me, I modified mine with a 10 speed stick shift from a semi truck and included the bigger engine from the truck too, it would top out at 90+.

So, one early morning while driving the empty bus on a quite empty freeway, en route to picking up a tour group, I was driving along at 60 in the number one lane (centermost lane) and saw a truck in front of me swerve into the shoulder. Then another, and wasn't sure what was going on. A few minutes later, a Ford sedan was right in front of me. THEN, he slammed on his brakes! I swerved to miss him, hit the air horn, cussed loudly, and I looped around him. Minutes later he was back in front of me. And slammed his brakes on again. Now it registered that he was likely trying to stage an accident so he would collect insurance. He had been unsuccessful with the earlier ones that I saw swerve miss him, so now he was trying me. Well, I went "Zero to Pissed off in 5 seconds" and decided to 'teach him a lesson'. I dropped the tranny a few gears, surprised him by chasing him down the freeway, and at about 70mph, I tapped his bumper a few times! No damage, not even a broken tail light for him. I was good at that sorta stuff, having worked a movie a few months before where I did some stunt driving in the bus so what the hell right?

He stopped on the side of the road, and apologized for causing me to swerve, said since there were no damages to his car, that things were OK. I suggested going to the Sheriff station and filing report. Nope, he said it was not necessary and left in his car. HOWEVER, in a year I got served with a $2 million lawsuit from him! He settled for $17,000 but in the 1980s that was good money, and apparently he did this a few times a year according to the insurance company! They found it was his way to make a good income, but for the insurance companies, they said it was cheaper to pay his settlements than it would be to fight million dollar lawsuits in court! UGH.

However, I realized in MY anger moment, had he done anything unexpectedly as I was tapping his bumper at 70 mph, my 50,000 pound vehicle could have rolled over his car and killed him! And I would have messed up my life, my future and done him a number too!

I carried a LOT of anger for many reasons before I started to realize where some of that anger came from. Over time, I've dealt with much of it, and at least realized how pissed I was having to give up being a kid, having my own sexuality issues in a time when it was not okay, being an only child married at 6 to my mother, dad being an absent father while physically present! Etc, etc.

———⁂———

Aunt Lil

My Journey to Self, recognizing the roles that my parents had failed in, realizing I had missed out being a kid, coming to grips with being an Adult Child who need to have a childhood at some point, was enhanced, aided and prodded by Aunt Lil who just died this past year at 100 yrs of age! Aunt Lil was the ONLY relative, so became 'THE' one even though we were not close. BUT she ended up being very important in my journey to SELF.

As usual, I have to give a shortish aside about Aunt Lil before sharing how she helped my Journey to Self. Lil was Lil, a victim of the world in her mind. There were many who knew her, and respected her, but not a lot of love for her since she had a hard time giving love. I use the example of this type of person that she was, and most of us have one or two in our lives, but IF, on one of my many flights to Europe or across the US, my plane had crashed and Lil got the call that "Jimmy died in the crash" her response would be tears for 15 minutes for Jimmy... THEN, "Why does this always happen to me, my only child died at 42, my two husbands died, my four dogs all died, and now Jimmy dies. Why me? Why does this happen to me?" Madame Victim expounds on her victimness!

On well, now back to my infamous year 2000 Millennium Christmas and New Year's. And wasn't welcoming in the year 2000 more of a snore than we had expected? Crap, 2020 turned out to be THE DRAMATIC type of stuff we had awaited in 2000 that didn't happen. But for 2000, I went east for my annual holiday trip. Visiting my 'adopted/extended' family, the family that came with my relationship. Even though my partner Ross had died 7 years before 2000, his family and I had stayed close and have continued to this day. His mother, became a surrogate mother for me, and his brother and sister, and their spouses and children have become the family contact I missed as a kid and for my first 45 years of life. On that trip East in 2000, I had some free time and rode down to Nutley, N.J. where my only surviving natural blood relative lived. Dear Aunt Lillian. I had no real interest in seeing her personally. As a kid I had heard a lot of negative stuff about her and her kid, my cousin, from my mother. She was actually not a blood relative, but her husband was my father's older brother and thus a real relative. While they were my only aunt, uncle and cousin when I was growing up, outside of my paternal grandmother who made no bones about not really caring for me, they were THE family. Limited, yes, but family officially.

Over the years, my mother reminded me constantly that my Aunt, Uncle and their son, my cousin Bobby, were losers, and we stayed as distant as we could. We visited only as needed a couple of times a year even though we lived only about an hour away. AND, as noted later in this section, I realized much later in my life, that Mother's reasoning for that was based on her controlling me, my life, keeping us 'married emotionally' and so I wouldn't find out some truths about HER life that might have changed our 'loving fucked up emotional marriage'. Sadly, some of my most fond childhood memories were with my Uncle Sam (he died in '58), and often with cousin Bobby along too, when he would take me to see and ride trains. Sam was the only relative/role model so special to me, a sanctuary for me. I didn't realize how much he meant to me at the time. I was a mechanical nerd, fascinated with things like big trucks, buses, airplanes. And, boy did I love trains, and Uncle Sam was an avid train fan, and he loved to take pictures of them. In New Jersey, trains were a main mode of transportation and still are today. We lived only houses away from a railroad station that had trains that ran to NYC which we took often. I would stand on the bridge over the tracks and watch often. I knew what each model of locomotive was and Uncle Sam and I would compare notes on the different engines when we were together. Cousin Bobby didn't really give a damn about much about anything but Cousin Bobby, so Uncle Sam enjoyed it when I was around.

Uncle Sam had a home movie camera, the precursor to today's video cameras. They were 8mm film cameras. He would film the trains - old steam engines, early diesels, live action - and then show them to us at the holidays. A treat for me. Of course, he also filmed every Christmas gathering and birthday. One of his favs was getting filmed as he dragged in the freshly cut Christmas tree every year. He'd bring it up the steps into the living room for the annual adventure of trimming the tree! Today we can all take videos with no effort, then we had to take the film from the camera, go to a camera processing place, leave the film and a few days or week later, go back and pay $$ to get it. But that was then, and now as an adult, I am still a train buff, and have been buying commercially available video's of the old trains as well as go for rides on trains when I can.

Well, many times over the years after we moved from New Jersey to go out west, I had thought about Uncle Sam's movies and really wanted to see them. I had lost contact with my Aunt. She had had a difficult time. After Uncle Sam died, then she eventually met another man who seemed to be a great guy. They got married, and he had been dealing with cancer. He died after just 5 years together. And to top things off, her son, my cousin, died mysteriously in their home a few years later. Suicide or murder, it was not truly resolved. Sad. Bobby was likely gay, but then it was so NOT okay to be gay. He tended to date married women, a clue that he might be gay! Got very involved with a gal who was married to a Sargent in the local police depart. It was a small department, and he was warned to stay away from this lady. One day, Aunt Lil was at the shore, getting ready to head back to their city home, and yes, at 41 years of age, Bobby still lived at home with mother, when she got a call from city neighbor that she should head home to deal with issue. When she arrived, she found out Bobby had been shot, local police said it was suicide, no investigation needed. He lasted 12 hrs and expired in hospital without regaining consciousness. They found a pistol in his room and a bottle of tranquilizers so it was written up as depression caused suicide.

Side light again, 20+ years later, when I was back in Aunt Lil's life, she asked me to go into Bobby's room which she had not been in since he died. She had gone in, cleaned the blood up when she got home that fateful day, and closed the door. No one was allowed in the room until she asked me one day, now that she trusted me and we had gotten close, to take care of something in the the room. I found the infamous bottle of tranquilizers that concluded the investigation by the police - it was a bottle of 25 pills, that had been filled at the pharmacy, 7 years before the time of his death. AND, there were still 12 pills left. So had only used 13 pills in 7 years - doesn't sound like major depression to me. PLUS, the gun was removed from the house by the police and destroyed. Interestingly, that gun was an antique pistol that Uncle Sam found when he was in South America in the 1930's working on a project. Theoretically, it had not been fired since 1930 or before. Sam and Bobby weren't into shooting, so it just sat in the drawer for all those years. Hmm, did it really get used by Bobby, or could the police decided he was done with his wife having an affair with Bobby? At the time, I understand when it was brought up as an issue, Aunt Lil was told that it was a closed case, no need for any investigation. Oh well.

Over the years, for about 25 years on the West Coast, I heard occasionally through my estranged mother cryptic updates regarding Aunt Lil and her life. We never traveled East to see them. My father did not ever contact his nephew Bobby, or his sister-in-law, Lil. I did try writing to her regarding the old train movies about once a year. I really wanted to see them and see if she would let me get them copied for my viewing. And when I was settled in with my partner Ross, who was from New Jersey, so now that we were traveling East to see his, now "our family", it was the ideal time to pick up the movies so I could see them. I had no real interest in seeing Aunt Lil, just accessing the movies.

So, I wrote her a number of times, and got no response. However, after writing for years to her, on my fateful trip to New Jersey for the 2000 Millennium New Year's and Christmas Holiday, I drove through her neighborhood on my way to attend my "extended/ chosen" in-laws for a New Years Day get-together. Aunt Lil was living back in the house she and her first husband, my train lovin' Uncle Sam had owned and bought 55 years before. She kept it all along while she was married to the other guy who died after 5 years. Confused yet? Sorry.

But I had had some really nice moments and positive memories as a kid watching Uncle Sam running his train layout in the basement of that house. He was an architect wanna be, like my father had been, but in his case his father pushed him into practical work, he did as dad told him, so Uncle Sam used his smarts to be an accountant. Damn by the time he died in 1958 he was pulling in about $65 a week and all the eggs he wanted from the egg farm he did the accounting for! What could be better in life?

There were warm memories of that house. Uncle Sam used those architect thought processes to design the most cool model train set up in the basement. Around the perimeter of the basement, at about 4 feet from the floor was a narrow ledge, about 4 inches wide, due to the way the cinder blocks had been set for the house. He utilized that ledge all the way around the basement to put train tracks, and in one corner was the model railroad terminal where the trains were stored when they were not running around. At another spot was a little town, and another a mountain and lake scene, etc. Totally cool. With parallel train tracks it was great too, to have races of trains. For me a dream. Ironically, his own son Bobbie had no interest in trains, but when I would visit it was awesome. And it provided an escape for Uncle Sam to go into his basement and work on 'Sam's Miniature World'. Nice.

Too, for me, in those kid days, it was cool just being there with relatives. So, in the year, 2000, thanks to the ubiquitous cell phones that were becoming the norm, I drove by her house. In the drive way was a gold Ford Crown Victoria sedan. A good sign, Aunt Lil was old, and damn, what other than a Buick would be a more indicative car that an older person lived there!

I went to a local donut shop two blocks away, did some thinking, got a bit emotional and teary thinking of the kid days there, and Uncle Sam. I missed him, and remembered that when he died in 1959, I had really cried. He had gone to vote, it was the year JFK ran for office, Lil said he came home from voting with major indigestion and heart burn, went upstairs in their house for Alka Seltzer and dropped dead in front of the medicine cabinet. He was cool, at my 8th grade graduation where I was the embarrassed kid from all the 'mother drama' bullying, and humiliation I had gone through, when my name was called in the class of 400 students, Uncle Sam stood up and yelled, "That's my nephew!". Nice.

After sitting there eating another 'comfort food donut' or two, I dialed 411 and got her phone number! The phone rang, and Aunt Lil answered. 'Hello, Aunt Lillian, this is Jimmy, a voice from the past, your nephew'. She got quiet, and was hesitant about talking and visiting, and had many caveats about why we couldn't get together. She mentioned that my letters about the train movies were still sitting around on her desk for the past years. Eventually, she said, 'Look, how about stopping by for just about 15 minutes. I have a cold, so normally I'm with my family (from her mother's side no connection to my father nor me) on New Years, but I was too sick today to go'. I drove back up to her house, apprehensive about the visit. Crap, it had been 40 years since I had seen Aunt Lil, 40 years since I had last been to that house for my Uncle's funeral. 30 years since I had sent or received even a Christmas card from her, and now, what to expect?

In my mind, all I really wanted were the damn movies and to be on my way. Im thinking, please, skip the small talk, let me find out about the movies and get on my way to more important things and get to Ross' family in Plainfield, just 20 minutes away, and our New Year's Day celebration. That New Year's Eve, (remember it was the millenium 2000) so I had spent it in the infamous New York Time's Square, the ultimate way to do New Year's in my mind. Now today was just an anti-climax. So I wanted to keep it short and sweet.

I kept thinking what had Aunt Lil to offer? According to what I had heard as a kid from my mother - very little. My mother had very few positive words about Aunt Lil, or even Uncle Sam when I was growing up. They had just "come with the marriage" since my father and Sam were brothers and Lil was even more distant since she was only involved by marriage. As per my mother, not much to talk about, not much to offer.

Well, our 15 minute visit turned into 4 hours! And for once in my life, I didn't say much. And for those who know me, that alone is amazing. Aunt Lil did most of the talking, and boy did she. It was great! I was hearing things about our families and things about my kiddom (i.e., childhood) that were great connections and "aha's" about stuff that I'd wondered about as a kid. Having had virtually no family other than my mother and father - who never wanted to talk about our family, extended family, or even their own early years - it was so exciting for me to hear about people who were part of my past, and even about myself as a baby, and as a kid growing up! Growing up, I had heard "zip" as a kid about my mother and father's earlier lives; or even about their times together before marriage; the marriage and the reasons for it; the activities when I was an infant and little kid. They were mum about their pasts and little said about about my birth and our early lives.

Now listening to Aunt Lil, I heard lots! As I listened it felt great and grounded me a lot, finally finding and understanding who Little Jimmy was. I had always had clues about stuff, but Lil verified so much. She gave a somewhat startling confirmation that my mother had been married prior to my father. Something I had suspected when I was 10 and found an old Social Security Card with my mother's first name but a different last name. When I asked my mother back then about it, she had quickly informed me it was just a card she got for a stage name she was gonna use if she got to be a dancer with the Rockette's which she had wanted to do. The name on the card was Marion Brugger, didn't seem like much of a stage name to me! Brugger? No, something short and non-ethnic would have sounded much more appropriate. For instance like my great Aunt who had been a performer, changed her name from Blanche Parsocouta, to Blanco Parks for performing. Now that was a stage name, not Brugger particularly during World War 2 era when Germany was our enemy. So I always suspected something even as a kid.

Aunt Lil, talked about how she and my mother had been such close friends, and buddies before either of them got married. That they had lived together in an apartment, done the young career woman stuff together banging around the city (Newark, NJ and New York City which are just across the river from each other), surviving their 20's. They even worked together at different points in the same companies. Then the bombshell from Aunt Lil, "Your mom and Bud, her first husband, seemed to be getting along so well, everybody liked Bud, he was such a nice guy. It was a surprise when Marian announced she was gonna divorce Bud and marry Jim. You knew your mother was married before didn't you? Bud was such a nice guy, I wonder what happened to him. Well all of a sudden your mother divorced Bud, and a few weeks later she married my Sam's brother, your dad, Jim."

Wow. HAPPY NEW YEAR!!! Yes, I had assumed my mother had been married before my father, but she never had confirmed it. Nor would my father confirm or talk about it, his standard answer to most stuff when I was growing up and to this question about whether she had been married before was "Ask your mother."

Wow. She really was married, divorced and re-married!! But, upon thinking, the time line for the divorce and re-marriage. Wait, that was too short of a time to get a divorce, even today, a few weeks doesn't do it. So, did she just lie? Oh, gosh what a shock that my dear sainted mother would ever lie! Oh yeah, that's right, yes, there were those little "white lies" she always talked about. Yes, she'd point that there IS a difference between lying versus just not telling the truth. AA folks say that "Alcoholics never lie, they just don't always tell the truth". Lying is pre-meditated, versus not telling the truth which is done to protect someone's feelings, yeah sure, WHATEVER!!! And with Alcoholics, they DO believe they can stop drinking whenever they want, and that they KNOW their limits. YUP. Uh huh. So, where does this marriage situation fit in? Fudging a bit, lying, stretching the truth, wanting to not hurt anyone's feelings...or just fucked up? Hmm, I'll go for the last at this point.

Now, take a moment, and let's think it through. Since I was born a year and a half after her marriage to Jim, and inspite of that bitch Grandma's accusation that with my blue eyes and blond hair that I couldn't be a real Gordon - Grandma missed that class about blue eyes and recessive gene's, huh - well, in spite of her wish that I wasn't, the physical look is there that I am a Gordon, as in my father's child, BUT the kick is that after being called a Bastard for various reason's in my life more than once, I guess I can own that legally now and be a legitimate Bastard because there ain't no way, my mother got a divorce - a legally accepted and recognized one at least - in the time frame that occurred between her leaving her first husband, Bud and marrying my father, Big Jim! So she and my father, probably were never legally married and were living in sin, as per the church, for the 44 years they were together! No wonder she didn't want me to ever hang out with or talk to Aunt Lil before! At the end of the 4 hours, I had to excuse myself and go. I was drained, but in a good way.

After all this input, now I was not going to continue my journey to my partner's family outing. I went out to the car, drove a few blocks, pulled into an empty parking lot, somewhat stunned. I called a few friends out in California, and cried a bit. I now was beginning to find more out about me, to hear that I did have a bit of a childhood, and in a way, I realized that my mother, and father were more screwed up than I had imagined. Or better, it had really confirmed some of my thoughts. Part of that was very healthy, because it was confirming that I wasn't just reading things into my life, but that they were real things. That things had been fucked up in many ways.

I was an emotional wreck by this point, and what was even more disturbing, was to find out that Aunt Lil was a cool lady! (To meet this person that I had preconceived notions about, how did I feel, the injustice of not enjoying her for 40 years Lil said that too) Wow. Sweet. I felt a real bond and in some ways, that was really disturbing. I had been lead to believe she was a total loser, and surprise, over the last 15 years my dear mother had done a good job of convincing Lil that I was the proverbial loser and creep too. My mother had told Aunt Lil, "You'd never recognize Jimmy now, he is really old, fat and bald", sweet words from a loving mother who told Aunt Lil this is what she had seen when her son(ME) did the

Montel Williams TV talk show as the guest shrink and some other TV shows in the 1990s.

Dammit mother Marian, so much for being able to be a proud mom and happy your kid was doing well!! But instead making me out to be crap with your salacious lies and back stories to get me fired, or have folks be afraid of me.

Wow, what weirdness Aunt Lil's visit was for me that fateful day. Finding this person, Aunt Lil, who actually knew me as an infant, and as a little kid, in many ways better than I knew myself. And who was a nice, gentle soul type person. She was not angry, not hostile, not bitter as my mother always painted a verbal picture of Lil. Wow, after losing two husband's and her only child to death, to not be bitter, that is amazing. She's managing life gracefully. Not in denial, but accepting that life deals weird and bad blows at times, and isn't always fair, but that it goes on. A gentle soul still trying to enjoy today, and to enjoy the people who are alive. What a nice experience for me to balance my own mother's bitterness and hatred for life. I knew then I had to go back soon and see Aunt Lil, and share time with her. When I got back out west, I wrote Lil and said I'd be back a.s.a.p.

In the spring, I had the chance. A comedienne friend Ellen was doing a road tour around the US of stand-up comedy, starting on the East coast. It would last about two months, ending back up on the East coast. This was a perfect excuse for me to fly east, and spend some more time with Aunt Lil, and catch a few of my friend's road shows. So, I flew back, stayed with my "mother-in-law" Muff, ran around to Atlantic City and New Brunswick, NJ for Ellen's shows. A whirlwind visit!

On that trip, Aunt Lil and I visited a number of days. I had a great time. The weekend that we were going to ELLEN's Atlantic City show. It started out with a drive up to Bloomfield with Aunt Lil to see the old house where I lived when I was brought home from the hospital after being born. Eerie in a way. And there was "an energy" that came up for me, as we drove around there - negative and creepy, but it was present. We only lived there a year with my bitchy Grandmother Gordon, before we moved to the Jersey Shore. Later I had spent time as an older child in that area when my mother and I would visit my Grandmother Gordon. She had moved out of her old house, but stayed in the same city. We had moved to the shore when I was only about a year old so I didn't really know the house, but visiting later we had spent time there before heading West.

Now, I felt more connected to 'me'. Perhaps in a Shirley McClaineish way but connected nonetheless. Actress Shirley was a bit esoteric, "I don't need anyone to rectify my existence. The most profound relationship we will ever have is the one with ourselves." So yes, I connected to Lil, connected to Jersey, connected a bit to little Jimmy and things that related to "little Jimmy". Things were making some sense. Lil and I rode around to some of the later places my grandmother Gordon lived My mother and I had my final trip to see Grandma at her place the day she had a stroke when we moved West. We were there when the ambulance guys removed her to the hospital. OH my, Memories - good and bad and weird and odd, but memories.

They say "you can't go back", but today, as a shrink, I strongly advocate "going back", riding/ walking around in areas where you grew up, spending time in the old place. Feel the feelings. Hell, those places contributed to who you are now, helped make you who, and what, you are today. The good memories, as well as the shitty one's. They will all come up in you head when you make a visit. So go, process them out. Some of the crappy ones will get worked out now, years later and free you. And some you will be stuck with but have more understanding of what its all about!

Well that weekend, eventually Lil and I ended up at Ellen's show in Atlantic City. We had a great time, and later that night, too soon, the weekend with Aunt Lil was over.

Again, as I drove away after dropping Lil back a her North Jersey home, I was listening to some great music on the car stereo, and the tears flowed a bit. Partly in happiness to have re-connected with Lil and partly in recognizing that we are both much older now, and wondering if we will get to spend much time, enough time together. Feeling a bit cheated that I had missed out on this connection for the past 40 years. And feeling partly in mourning for that little Jimmy who now through Aunt Lil, I was getting to know better. Yes, thank you actress Shirley MacLaine for introducing me to think more outside the box too. Yes, getting to know me, and learning about some of the things I had missed about 'myself' while growing up. As a child of alcoholics, I quickly had to become an adult, the 'I never got to be a little boy' part of this story. Partly in feeling pissed at mother for lying about so much. Partly bitter too, but strongly thinking there has to be another visit back to Jersey, soon! And there was right up 'til Lil died at 100, and my partner's mother Muff died at 90. Thank you both for helping complete me in many ways, not that I am complete or any of are TOTALLY COMPLETE, but filling in some of the gaps and helping me define ME.

HEALING STARTS???

And now is a good time to point out that both Aunt Lil and my mo-in-law, Muff, became two of my "healthy parents". Surrogate parents, along with an older friend, Shirley. They provided the most healthy parenting I got in my life, plus the years with my partner Ross who was so honest, strong and became my first really "healthy parent" before Muff, Aunt Lil and Shirley came on board. Thank you Ross, Lil, Shirley and Muff for what you did for me. Thank you. Healthy parents want what is best for YOU, not just for themselves, not controlling you to be there only for them and meet their needs, BUT what is best for you even if it doesn't meet their need at the moment!

From my book "9 Steps to a Better Life", also available on AMAZON/KINDLE, "When you were born, you had to rely on your parents for direction, care, feeding, security, safety. Basically everything. As you got older, other 'parent figures' came into your life too. These could be your teachers, Sunday School teachers, grandparents, little league coaches, television and movie characters, friends." AND for some of us, unexpected unofficial Surrogate Parents like mine listed above, who, even thought I was an adult at the time, they also parented me, as they told and suggested to me what I should do, could do, but unlike my mother, they supported me honestly in my goals for my sake NOT to meet their needs alone! Each was a gift of the type of gift that doesn't stop giving.

❑ ❑ ❑ ❑

Little Jimmy's Early Years

My mother's grandfather, the priest, Father John Parscouta, I mentioned, had been fortunate enough to be given a few perk's as a priest - including a summer bungalow at the "shore", Laurence Harbor, NJ. The word shore is beach to the rest of the world. Jersey Shore bungalows were primarily designed to be used in the summer, very spartan, unheated, not fancy. This shore place was a marriage present to Marian from her grandfather, and now her new husband and she would winterize it for full time living. It was two houses from the beach (150 feet or so), on the saltwater bay that was the entrance to New York Harbor. In the 20's, 30's and 40's. the little town was a hot spot for bathers and beach revelers. It had a nice a pier jetting out into the bay and a Dance Hall on the water front. By the 1950's, it was a somewhat financially depressed spot but provided a haven for new families to raise their kids. The bungalows got turned into homes, the cabana's that had lined the beach on the waterfront disappeared during a few hurricanes and it was now a year-round town, not just a summer retreat. Schools were enlarged, folks moved in and stayed full time as we did.

In the late '40s and 1950's the bay was getting pretty much polluted - along with many of the residents, as in depressed people who drank a lot! Up one of the rivers that fed our bay before it opened into the Atlantic Ocean, there was a company that made lead for paint, and yes, they used the river to cool their equipment, flush their plant, and dropped that waste into the River! Oh yeah, there was a cyanide plant up river, for whatever cyanide is produced for and they too shared their waste with the river.

And then there were the wonderful oil refineries located around our bay in Perth Amboy, convenient access to the ocean, so tankers could bring their crude oil from foreign shores, into Jersey to be refined and used by citizens all over this wonderful continent. And, there were occasional oil spills from those refineries, or from the ships themselves, and small accidents that added pollutants to the bay. As well, what better place to dump the holding tanks for the ship's onboard toilets and sewage system, than the river and bay. After all it just runs a little further east, to that vast waste dump, the ocean. Right? But maybe deposit some of the pollutants in the sand on the bay beaches on the way to that ocean!

Wow, today we know so much more about pollution, and learn about how we had kissed off our environment then. As I mentioned somewhere else in this book, God, who created the earth, must be sittin' up there at times, with her head in her hands, tears in her eyes, saying... "I gave you such a wonderful, beautiful, intricate playground, and look what you're doing to it."

As a little kid, I learned to swim amid dead jelly fish, dead mackerel, and upturned dying horseshoe crabs. Horseshoe crabs, these little helmet shaped creatures who had survived thousands of years intact, looking just as they did in prehistoric times until they met the Jersey shore! It did make fishing easier, because the fish glowed at night and were easier to see!! When a blood chemical analysis was done of my system by a doctor in California when I was in my 40's, my doctor noted a number of chemicals that had higher numbers, but wrote it off to, "Oh yeah, that's right, you were raised in Jersey." Is some kind of cancer somewhere around the corner in my future? Or did I build up high immunity to stuff from all the exposure? We'll see in time, we'll see in time. So far so good at 70.

I didn't enjoy the neighborhood kids, I hung out with a 70 yr old lady at the shore. Continuing my journey of never being a little boy, when I was 13, and we had moved to Arizona where my mother had been offered a job transfer with the Civil Service are of the Army. As a shrink, I would have to say that she would have made her dead mother, my demented Nanny who never knew who 'that kid(me) was when she came to visit', very proud, why? Because Marian was still a secretary, just what her mom wanted, not that horrible dancer or actress Marian had wanted to be, but a basic functioning secretary, a 'proper role for a woman' in Nanny's day. Not a whore actress or performer that Nanny felt her three sisters had become on Broadway. Well, she was not just a secretary but one working for the federal government in an office of military men, with ranks from Sargent to Colonel, six guys who were supervising a major government project - the development of unmanned spy planes - brought about by the infamous U-2 spy incident during Eisenhower's term when one of them was shot down over Russia. A number of aeronautical companies had been given contracts to develop, test and bring to production, "drones" - unmanned spy planes - that could do what the U-2 had done but with out the human weakness of telling the Russians about the project vs a mechanical drone that would NOT react to the threat of torture and death, and spill the beans of what the USA was doing.

And cute, perky, smart Marian was the only civilian in the office, and as the secretary, she was the office coordinator for this military contingent that was being sent to oversee and co-ordinate the three different companies that were awarded contracts for the drones. Thus even as a the lowly paid secretary, but the only civilian in the office she was important. So when it was time to send this team off to Arizona, to the infamous Yuma Army Test Station, civilian, civil service, Marian went as part of the package. It was good bye to friends, and the last of the living family, Aunt Lillian (her husband, my father's brother - Sam had died of a stroke on election night two years before), her son and the paternal grandmother who recently had that stroke I mentioned and was convalescing. Big Jim had had little contact with his mother, so her stroke was no big issue for him. He and I became busy making the arrangements for the family to move to

Arizona. Jim felt his mother would just have to take care of her self. As it turns out, Aunt Lillian became the pawn here, and though she was related only by marriage to Grandma, remember this was the "loving" bitch who had pushed little me off her lap and rejected me when I was 6, Aunt Lil was left to take good care of Grandma, while Grandma's own son, big Jim packed up, moved to Arizona and ignored her. And little ACOA Jimmy took on the packing at responsibility cuz big Jim (remember I never called him father, or dad but Jim from the time I was about 4) was busy still at his store and important customer to his local tavern.

After we arrived in Yuma, Arizona and set up home, Grandma Gordon rebounded quickly from her stroke back in New Jersey, surprising every one, and she was able to get up and get around again in no time. She wrote to her son, my father, over and over. He ignored her as he had always done, and I remember well, my mother and I did the letter writing to her to kept contact. All this while Big Jim did more important things, like drink himself into oblivion, or go rock hunting on the Yuma desert, then, oh yeah, drink himself into oblivion again.

When Jim's mother got really sick again, and was expected to die a years later after we had left Arizona, Big Jim who had taken an offer by the military to 'get outta town', since he was a federal government employee too, and was working then on a project for them in Guam. Many guys liked taking positions like that to get away from issues at home. So, with his mother terminal, the government was willing to pay for his flight to the East Coast to see his mother before she died. But, in his usual, sensitive, loving way - fueled by passive aggressive behavior - he turned it down and said he could do her no good! Gallant, he stayed on working in Guam, doing his job for the government, oh yeah, and shacking up with girlfriend there who was married to one of his team working partners in Guam. Handy. Convenient.

In the years that it had now been since the family and I had moved out West, and that Grandma had had her stroke, her son - Big Jim - had never called and talked to her, nor written her a letter. Letter after letter arrived from her, addressed to him and then from Aunt Lil, begging him to write her. Finally, five years later he sat down and wrote her a short note. Guess what? Aunt Lil called and said Grandma died within a week of getting that letter. Satisfied finally to hear from him? Or just in shock to hear from him? Either way, she was dead. Not a big loss to humanity. She was never a very loving, caring, sharing person. Her nick name coined by her "nearest and dearest" friends was "ol' hatchet face".

Yes, going back a little in my story, we did only stay in Yuma for the 3 years of the contract as mentioned earlier. BUT during that time we lived there, I took on even more responsibilities as the ADULT CHILD of ALCOHOLICS (ACOA). We tried a few different homes in Yuma, including a new design concept classic 3 bedroom 2 bath ranch style tract home that utilized ONLY aluminum foil in the outside walls for insulation from the Yuma scorching summer heat that often hit 115 to 120 degrees. LOGIC of the architect of the tract was we didn't need to waste wads of 4 inch to 6 inch thick fiberglass insulation like many homes had in country since Yuma didn't have super cold winters, had at least limited sun 300+ days a year, and aluminum foil is all that was needed to reflect the heat from the sun. WRONG! On the few days it hit 30 degrees during the night, we were very cold AND the head came in so badly from June til October, we had thick dark drapes up, two rows on each window and it was miserable inside.

So, after renting another house, we ended up in the Country Club Mobile Park which catered to Snow Birds, i.e., folks who came to the desert in the winter from very cold places like all over Canada, Montana, Idaho... There were only about 12 full time families in that place, the other 80 or so units were the snowbirds. BUT I AGED a lot! Why? Cuz it was an upscale type of place in a way where the snowbirds were well off enough to have homes up north, then winter places in Arizona. I met doctors, lawyers, biz folks and dentists as I would be like any other Senior Citizen there (though I was 14-16 at the time!) play lots of Shuffleboard, lawn bowling, cards and very good at Pot Luck dinners with Bingo! It was nice being a super nerd like I was, and I got some great interactions from these folks as we'd sit and talk back and forth and I learned so much about life. And death since so many were on their last legs.

BUT, little Jimmy also got some more ACOA stuff in Yuma, when at 15 years of age, after hearing mother complain constantly about big Jim, I went to an attorney and got things set up for a divorce for her. Yup, I looked older started having to shave at 15 - in those days we couldn't have mustaches or any form of beard. I was taken into the principals office at 15 when I was a Junior in high school, handed an electric shaver and told to shave.

So, yes, I sorted things out, and convinced my mother it was something she might do since she whined about it all the time. She did go to the attorney but backed out. But little Jimmy had been the good "adult" again and had the paperwork ready if she wanted to do it.

There were many other adult things I did while in Yuma, including getting drivers license at 15½ and having Thelma Schwartz ask me to help her out. Her grand daughter was flying in from Chicago for the summer, and would I drive with her hubby to Phoenix airport to get the grand daughter with her hubby. They lived there full time, he was a retired car designer, she had just had some surgery so couldn't make the 6 hr, 360 mile round trip so I could drive oneway and her hubby Frank would drive back. On my for a car nerd what could be better. He a brand new high end red and white Oldsmobile station wagon that had some extra modifications and moved out well. I had just started driving and this would be one of my first long drives. Arizona had only "Reasonable and Prudent" for speed limits on long highways. Two lane highways were the norm, only highway 80, now Interstate 8, was mostly two lanes. I drove the speed most were driving, 80 mph, excited as hell. Then passed someone, when "OH CRAP, I misjudged this one" when I say another car coming towards us briskly. After all it was prolly one of my FIRST ever times of passing someone at 80! So was hitting 100 mph or more as we zipped by, got back into our own lane and didn't die in a head on crash. Hmmm, did it leave a memory? Hell yes if 50 years later as I write this book it was one of my strongest memories from Yuma! And, I did learn a lot quickly about how to judge distances driving. We picked up the grand kid, had lunch in Phoenix and after 390 miles of driving were back home, safely and in one piece, for dinner with Thelma.

Yuma taught me much, having been a suburban kid on the Jersey shore with NYC to go shopping, and after Yuma, for the rest of my life living in LA area both as suburban and city dweller I had Yuma's total rural life for comparison. It was good for the time, but not "me" and helped me decide where I wanted to settle.

❑ ❑ ❑ ❑

I DON'T WANT
YOU TO
    SAVE ME.
I WANT YOU TO
STAND BY
MY SIDE
    AS I SAVE
MYSELF.

III. WHAT I LEAVE FOR YOU READERS: "IT'S NEVER TO LATE FOR A HAPPY CHILDHOOD"

"Life, Liberty and the Pursuit of Anger" as was mentioned earlier was the original title of the book. It was to be in 3 parts and sort of ended up that way still. Part One tells what it is. Part Two talks abou the ANGER that came out, as I reviewed what brought me to recognize what was in me forever. Some of the 'who's' and their impact and relationship in my life, put some faces to the issue. Part Three, LIBERTY, is the freeing of one's self from the bondage to that parent, and dealing with your anger, repressed and overt, that Emotional Incest has caused.

Managing Life. It sounds trite we're always looking for a new way of saying the same old things. However, I think managing your life gracefully is a good concept. That infamous philosopher extraordinaire Rodney King, with his infamous post- Rodney King Riots statement in 1992 "can't we all just get along" put it well perhaps not realizing it.

Fulgum with his teaching "All I need to know I learned in Kindergarten", and Elton John singing the

Lion King song "Circle of life, there's more to see than can ever be seen, More to do than can ever be done... But the sun rolling high... Keeps great and small on the endless round
It's the circle of life, And it moves us all
Through despair and hope, Through faith and love,
'Til we find our place On the path unwinding."

All of those quotes say the same thing. The concept is some of us live life better than others no matter what cards we've been dealt.

Will we put in the life pretty much we tend to get out of it. My partner Ross and I traveled often, he died at only 29 of AIDS, but I insert a life analogy here. We traveled with leather duffel bags. We would stuff them to the max heading out on a trip, then throw them on the bed to unload at home. Life at times is like the duffel bags, the memories of the trip come up as the duffel bags get emptied. When we got home to take everything out of that bag that we used on the trip that we took with us on the trip that we brought back from the trip, and the leather duffel is now slouched or collapsed on the bed the duffel bag now just represents a quote "medium" for our travel and now the good feelings and the memories are all what's left of the trip.

When Ross died and I looked at him crumbled slumped on the bed and realized the life was gone out of him. That he was like the empty duffel bag. His life trip was over the trip was done. What we put into his life what he put into his life, what he and I got out of his life, what his family and everyone got out of his life were now left as memories.

Fill your LIFE's duffel bag to the MAX, enjoy today, yesterday and our concept of tomorrow. Look around, see, feel, sense ... LIVE.

WHAT were Miltowns:

They were my mother's pills of choice, the 1960's Addiction Med. Call your doctor, your pharmacy, go to other docs, and pharmacy's to get all you wanted. In that era there were no ONLINE records of meds so easy to just go to the next town over, see a doc, get a prescription and go to one of the multitude of local pharmacies, we had Sal's, Merv's, Circle Pharm. All maintained hand written records on site only!

Miltown was a suggested tablet to control anxiety, stress, nervousness. Actually suggested when trying to conceive to relax during intercourse. It's a potent little tranquilizer called Miltown, after Milltown, the New Jersey hamlet where it was manufactured in 1955. Despite virtually zero advertising, the release of the original "mother's little helper" set off a consumer stampede. By 1957, Americans had filled 36 million prescriptions for Miltown, more than a billion pills had been manufactured and these so-called "peace pills" accounted for one third of all prescriptions. The drug's popularity has fallen off a cliff since the 1960s, when studies found that it caused psychological dependence. But it nonetheless launched the age of psychiatric cure-alls. Dozens of "lifestyle drugs" (like Xanax and Paxil, which also treat anxiety) have followed in its wake, raising a perennial question: do we actually need these medications, or does Big Pharma push them on us?

IT'S A WRAP

I live and practice in the film and entertainment capital of the World, so as they say when they finish filming movie or winding up a night of a TV taping - "It's a Wrap." We are at the end of the book and our time together. A few years ago, I wrote a blog, that I will share here as part of 'my wrap.'

Finding about ourselves is a difficult journey, sometimes painful, and some never get 'there', but it can be wonderful in its own way. I'm sure you've heard the phrase psychological writers and 12 steppers toss about - "the Journey to Self." I have shared a lot of that with you in this book, and it fits so, so much in this context.

Make your Journey productive. Leave a legacy, impact many around you, and those who come after you. Too often someone says, 'If I can just help one person, I've done well', nope - that would be a waste of your talents, spread good things, teach many to sing, to dance, to enjoy, or even just to LOOK. Awe and wonder is the parent of the child inside of all of us, and the child is what keeps us humming... and singing... and dancing, when the adult in us is telling us NO. Listen to your kid.

Tonight I guess, as I sat here and watched "13" the movie and the emotions hit me as the young man was singing as he was doing his Bar Mitzvah, wrapping up his childhood and embarking on adulthood. The words that got me were, "I may be an adult now, but I think I have a little more homework to do and I just need a little more time to do it." YES even at my age, I get nervous because I hope to have a little more time to do a few more things, to leave a little more legacy, to help some more people. I don't know how much time I have, but I know that I have a lot less time in front of me than I do behind me. My dear partner died at age 29, so much time that should have been ahead, but he left me with a legacy that has influenced me. Everything I do has some inspiration 30 years later of what he instilled in me. I still "talk" him for support when I need.

In life we need to figure out some things as we go along, we get challenges, struggles and strife... but life would be so boring if we knew everything ahead of time wouldn't it? I have been blessed and cursed. There's some things I've done that if I knew what I know today I wouldn't of done, regrets, about things that I've done that were mistakes, but I overall have been so lucky to have been involved in people's lives, entertainment folks, International business people... And to have access to a home in Europe and feel like I'm a local in Paris, be a local in New York City/Jersey Shore area where I was raised AND a local out here in LA. I do take the time to stop and look.

IMPORTANT WORDS: "Stop, LOOK, Listen and Feel." There IS a world around us. There was an old Mama Cass song in the 80's, here is one clip from it that I've lived by for many years "Did you ever hold a child's hand to stop its trembling? Did you ever watch the sun desert the sky? Did you ever sit right down and have a cry? Friend, don't let the good life pass you by."

Use your talent. Make your journey worth it.

dr. g.

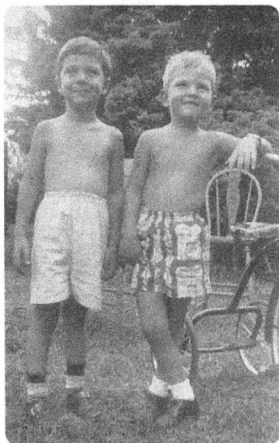

Memories...........

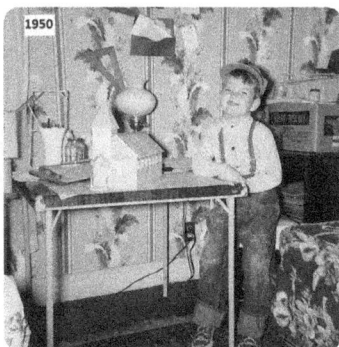

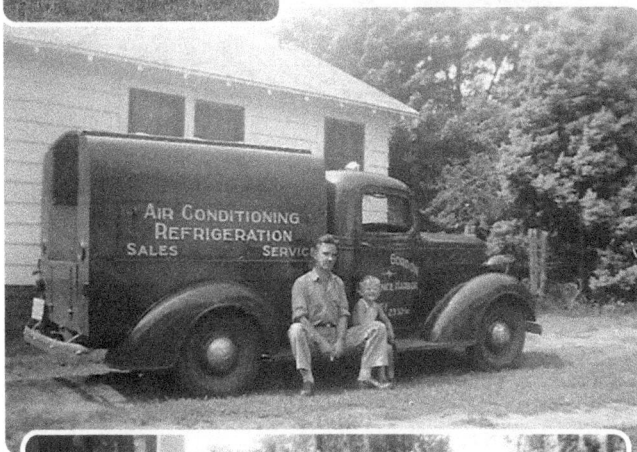

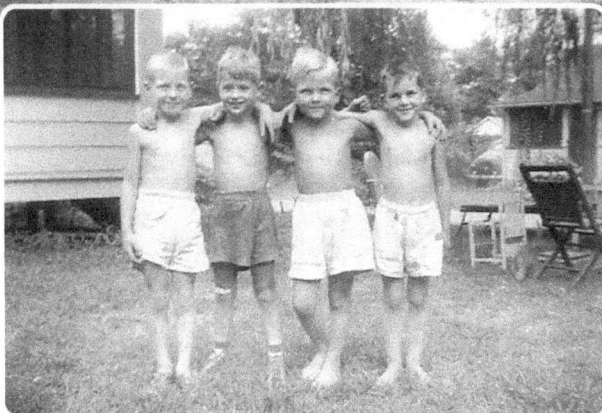

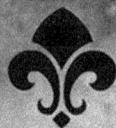

DO NOT EVER
APOLOGIZE FOR
THE MADNESS
WHICH MADE YOU
A
WARRIOR.

- Rune Lazuli

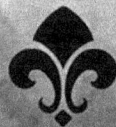

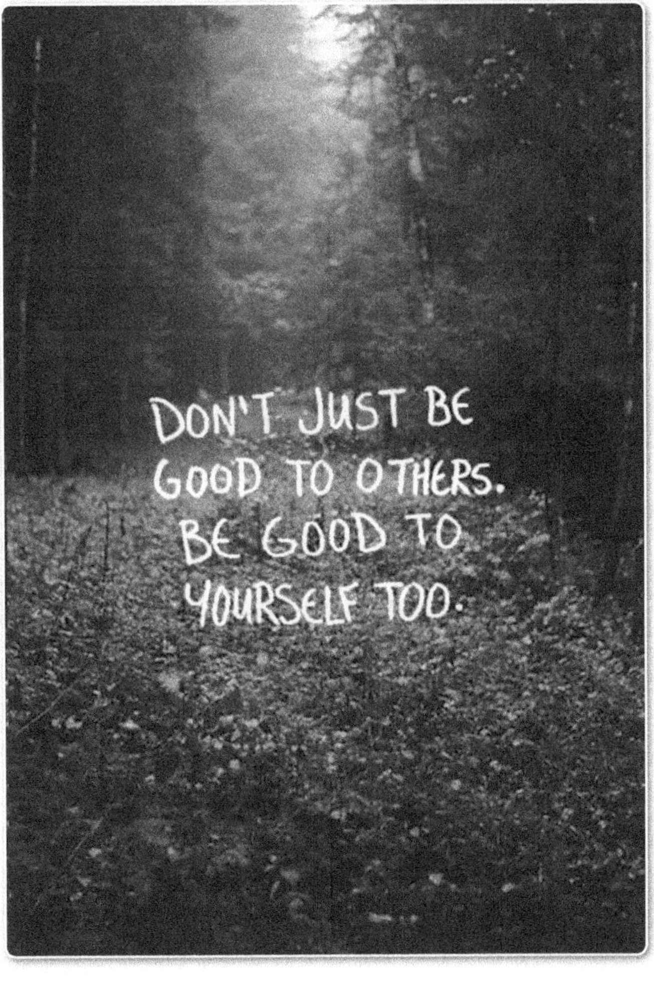
DON'T JUST BE
GOOD TO OTHERS.
BE GOOD TO
YOURSELF TOO.

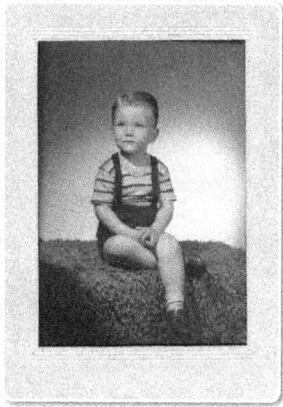

As Teddy Roosevelt told the kids in Newsies, I wish I could tell you I'll leave the world a perfect place, but all I can do is leave you with MORE tools, more awareness so you can have a better, fuller life...

dr g